Integrating Telemental Health Practice Into Counselor Education Training

HEATHER C. ROBERTSON

American Counseling Association
counseling.org

American Counseling Association
2461 Eisenhower Avenue, Suite 300
Alexandria, Viriginia 22314

Published in the United States of America

Library of Congress Cataloging-in-Publication Data

Names: Robertson, Heather C., author.
Title: Integrating telemental health practice into counselor education training / Heather C. Robertson.
Description: Alexandria, VA : American Counseling Association, [2025] | Includes bibliographical references and index.
Identifiers: LCCN 2024056565 (print) | LCCN 2024056566 (ebook) | ISBN 9781556204173 (paperback) | ISBN 9781394222872 (epub) | ISBN 9781394222889 (PDF)
Subjects: MESH: Distance Counseling--education | Counselors--education | Mental Health Teletherapy | Mental Health Services
Classification: LCC RA790.8 (print) | LCC RA790.8 (ebook) | NLM WM 18 | DDC 362.2071--dc23/eng/20250130
LC record available at https://lccn.loc.gov/2024056565
LC ebook record available at https://lccn.loc.gov/2024056566

Contents

Preface vii

Acknowledgements xi

Additional Contributors xiii

How to Use This Book

1. Understanding Telemental Health Practice 3
2. Teaching Telemental Health Practice 11

Foundational Counseling Curriculum

3. Professional Counseling Orientation and Ethical Practice 21
4. Social and Cultural Identities and Experiences 39
5. Lifespan Development 53
6. Career Development 69
7. Counseling Practice and Relationships 85
8. Group Work and Group Counseling 99
9. Assessment and Diagnostic Processes 113
10. Research and Program Evaluation 129

Entry-Level Specialized Practice Area

11. Addictions Counseling 145
12. Career Counseling 161
13. Clinical Mental Health Counseling 175
14. Clinical Rehabilitation Counseling 189

15. College and Student Affairs Counseling 205
16. Marriage, Couple, and Family Counseling 217
17. School Counseling 229

Other Considerations

18. Professional Practice and Fieldwork 247
19. Counselor Education and Supervision 255
20. The Future of Telemental Health Counseling and Training 269
Appendix A: ACA & NBCC Codes of Ethics on Telemental Health 279
References 287
Glossary 309
Index 315

Preface

My motivation to explore teaching telemental health came from an interaction with a student in 2015 while teaching a clinical mental health counseling internship class. The student was discussing her client's case and, at one point, remarked, "It's just hard because I see her on the VeeSee." My response to the student was, "What's the VeeSee?" panicking internally when the student explained that she was seeing her client via video conferencing software. I asked the student where she learned to counsel clients via videoconferencing and who was supervising her on that technology—because I knew it was not us.

Our program did not train students in what would come to be known as telemental health (TMH) in 2015, but this brief interaction alerted me that we should be. I took it upon myself to get trained. Having completed my master's degree in 1996 and my doctorate in 2010, I never received TMH training. Even though I remained in clinical practice, the agencies I worked with did not use TMH before COVID-19. I completed the distance credentialed counselor (DCC) training through Renewed Vision Counseling and became my institution's de facto TMH researcher and instructor. I later transitioned this credential to the Board Certified Telemental Health Provider (BC-TMH). I obtained grants in 2016 and 2018 focused on teaching TMH and my first book contract on the practice of TMH in 2019. Then, unexpectedly, in March of 2020, my prior training and research became of great importance as our students swiftly transitioned to digital delivery.

Digital delivery of counseling services, known as *telemental health*, is not new. Practices date back to the 1950s when psychiatrists conducted clinical interviews via closed-circuit television. Around 2000, technologies expanded through broadband internet and smartphones, opening digital counseling to a broader audience. Over the past 20+

years, a growing research base has verified its efficacy with multiple populations and clinical foci. In 2020, COVID-19 propelled the profession into widespread use of TMH, yet the training that prepared counselors for that transition is questionable. Some counselors may have transitioned to TMH with no training at all. Training in TMH, even before COVID-19, was problematic. No unified training standards exist for digital counseling delivery. Although there are national certification programs, these programs vary in terms of training content, cost, and length of time.

The training dilemma extends into counselor education programs. During COVID-19, the Council on the Accreditation of Counseling and Related Education Programs (CACREP) and state organizations approved the digital delivery of counseling services for fieldwork experiences. The newest 2024 CACREP standards do not specifically require counselor education programs to train students on TMH but do require training programs to address the "application of technology related to counseling" (CACREP, 2023, Standard 3.E.5) and for "establishing and maintaining counseling relationships across service delivery modalities" (Standard 3.E.7). Despite these directives, faculty may have limited knowledge or experience in the nuances of TMH delivery. There is a significant knowledge gap between those who were trained prior and those who will be trained in the future. Counselor educators training the next generation of counselors in digital delivery may lack knowledge and experience in TMH.

Even counselor educators trained in TMH practice can lack the tools to translate that knowledge into their training. Counseling curricula are already full of required information, and counselor educators and instructors may be unsure how to weave TMH content into their existing programs. Despite the growth, emergence, and increase of digital services, there are no resources on how an educator can provide training on TMH counseling. Various books have been written for practitioners on delivering TMH. Yet, to date, none exists for the educator or instructor charged with teaching TMH practice to counselors-in-training (CITs). This book addresses that shortcoming by providing a resource that counselor educators and instructors can use to train current and future counselors in TMH.

It should be noted that this book assumes that instructors hold a foundational knowledge of TMH practices. The book aims to support instructors in integrating TMH knowledge into their counselor education training programs. Instructors who lack foundational knowledge in TMH are encouraged to receive TMH training, review resources on

TMH, or engage in supervised TMH counseling prior to training counselors in TMH practice. Some suggested resources are provided in Chapter 1. The book is divided into four sections to support the integration of TMH concepts into counselor education.

Section 1 includes two chapters that set the stage for using the book within your curriculum. Chapter 1 provides general concepts on TMH and common definitions while also directing readers to additional resources for gaining TMH content knowledge. Instructors lacking knowledge or experience in TMH can start with the resources at the end of the chapter to develop that foundation. Chapter 2 discusses teaching TMH through a CACREP lens and multiple modalities such as on-campus, online synchronous, and online asynchronous. This chapter concludes with an introduction to *andragogy*, the practice of adult education, which informs the instructional delivery methods suggested.

Section 2 addresses the foundational CACREP curriculum, including Professional Orientation, Social and Cultural Diversity, Lifespan Development, Career Development, Counseling Practice and Relationships, Group Counseling and Group Work, Assessment and Diagnostic Processes, and Research and Program Evaluation. Section 3 addresses CACREP specialization areas, including Addictions, Career, Clinical Mental Health, Clinical Rehabilitation, College and Student Affairs, Marriage/Couple/Family, and School Counseling. In Sections 2 and 3, the format of the chapters includes Key Concepts, Teaching Techniques, and Sample Lessons.

Key concepts address CACREP standards, and two to three additional focus areas are worthy of attention. All CACREP standards within the curricular area are reviewed, and specific suggestions for integrating TMH concepts are included in alignment with each standard. The additional focus areas provide instructors with information or reminders on TMH topics that warrant special attention or emphasis within the counseling curriculum. Teaching Techniques within each chapter outline 10 suggested activities that instructors can utilize to actively integrate TMH into their counseling curriculum. Each chapter in Sections 2 and 3 contains two Sample Lessons on teaching TMH within the foundational or specialization areas. Several professionals across multiple organizations and institutions have contributed, coauthored, edited, and supplemented these lessons to provide the reader with diverse ideas, styles, and mechanisms to teach TMH. The lessons include interactive classroom activities, case studies, and lecture topics that instructors can modify to suit their instruction and student needs.

Section 4 includes additional considerations for integrating TMH content into the counseling curriculum. Chapter 18 addresses Professional Practice and Fieldwork, and Chapter 19 addresses Counselor Education and Supervision. These chapters also address CACREP curricular standards and teaching techniques but do not include sample lessons. Finally, Chapter 20 addresses future trends in TMH counseling and training.

Counselors are no longer just sitting across from their clients and students in physical spaces but meeting their clients and students where they are through digital delivery. Teaching TMH practice to the next generation of counselors can be daunting, particularly for those not trained and experienced in its use or those unsure how to integrate their TMH knowledge into the classroom. Technology is constantly changing, improving, and innovating. As educators and instructors, we commit ourselves to remaining current in the emerging practices of the field. This book intends to support instructors by linking key elements of TMH and CACREP standards directly to the curricular areas in which they teach. I hope to make the prospect of teaching TMH less intimidating and, by doing so, help you avoid the internal panic I experienced back in 2015.

Be well, practice wisely, and thank you for being open to teaching TMH counseling ethically and effectively. Future counselors are counting on our ability to do so.

References

Council on the Accreditation of Counseling and Related Education Programs. (2023). *2024*

CACREP standards. https://www.cacrep.org/for-programs/

Acknowledgements

Thank you to the American Counseling Association (ACA) for supporting this project. I am particularly grateful to Christine Fruin, Tom Cadorette, and the ACA for their ongoing support, their patience, and their constant advocacy for the counseling profession. Thanks to my colleague, Dr. Michael Jones, for our initial collaborations and for providing my first training in distance counseling back in 2016 through Renewed Visions, which sparked my knowledge and passion for telemental health. I'm also grateful to the many colleagues who contributed lessons to support the book—their input and expertise are valued more than I can express.

The Department of Counselor Education at St. John's University deserves a special shout-out. My goodness, this dream team of coworkers and colleagues is a group I am so grateful for: Gina, James, Ming, Nouna, Qiana, Bob, Leo, and Zoya—thank you for loving this field and enjoying training our students as much as I do. You are a wonderful group to be surrounded by. Special thanks go to Michelle Schwab, a St. John's University Clinical Mental Health Counseling student and rising star who dedicated hours of her own time—beyond her graduate assistant position—to help edit and review the book, for which I am incredibly grateful.

The foundation of my soul, my world, and my existence is my family and friends. I get by with a bit of help from my friends (or a lot): my Scituate Sailors, SU Boland crew, and SJU confidants—you know who you are. You sustain me, and I thank you. My mom and my sisters always buoy my mental health, and without them, I would surely sink. Ben, I'm eternally grateful to you. I love you for being the glue that keeps me together, as well as our family. Ryan and Sam, continue to let your spirits soar. Your individual journeys inspire me, and I cherish watching you grow into the kind men that you are. I'm lucky to be your mother.

Additional Contributors

To the many colleagues who contributed lessons to this book, thank you for your contributions. Your ideas and insights will be incredibly valuable to readers.

Kami Ball Tran, MS, LPC-S, RPT-S, NCC

James Bethea, PhD, LMHC, CRC, St. John's University

Pamelia Brott, PhD, LPC, NCC, ACS

Claudette Brown-Smythe, PhD, LMHC, ACS, NCC, CRC, SUNY Brockport

Gina Cicco, EdD, LMHC, NCC, Certified School Counselor, St. John's University

Robert Eschenauer, PhD, LMHC, NCC, St. John's University

Leo Gonzalez, PhD, LMHC, NCC, St. John's University

John J. S. Harrichand, PhD, LPC-S, LMHC, NCC, ACS, University of Texas at San Antonio

Cameka Hazel, EdD, MHC-LP, New York Institute of Technology

Nouna Jalilzadeh, PhD, LMHC, NCC, St. John's University

Michael Jones, PhD, LPC-S, NCC, BC-TMH, University of the Cumberlands

Ming-hui Li, EdD, LMHC, LPC, St. John's University

Tyce Nadrich, PhD, LMHC, NCC, ACS, Mercer University

Joni O'Hagan, MSEd, St. John's University

Michelle Perepiczka, PhD, LMHC, LPC, RPT-S, ACS, NCC, University of Phoenix

Brittany L. Prioleau, PhD, LCMHC, NCC, Mercer University

Matthew R. Shupp, EdD, NCC, BC-TMH, ACS, LPC, Shippensburg University of Pennsylvania

Jessica L. Sniatecki, PhD, CRC, SUNY Brockport

Qiana Spellman, EdD, Certified School Counselor, St. John's University

How to Use This Book

1

Understanding Telemental Health Practice

To provide effective instruction on telemental health (TMH), counselor educators and instructors must understand the practice of TMH. This chapter broadly introduces TMH and directs the instructor to additional resources to expand their knowledge.

The practice of telemental health, while not new, has been growing rapidly since the onset of the COVID-19 pandemic in 2020. A report by the Substance Abuse and Mental Health Services Administration (SAMHSA) indicates that mental health telemedicine services more than tripled between 2015 and 2020 (22.2% to 68.7%), with the most significant increase occurring between 2019 and 2020 (38% to 68.7%). Similarly, telemedicine services for substance use, which had seen little increase between 2015 and 2019, more than doubled between 2019 and 2020 (25.7% to 58.6%; Alvarado, 2021). Consumer awareness of TMH is also growing. In a 2021 survey by the American Psychiatric Association (APA), 60% of respondents indicated that they would use telemedicine for mental health care. Respondents who would use TMH increased from 49% in 2020 to 59% in 2021, with 66% of respondents ages 18–29 responding that they would utilize TMH services (APA, 2021). While the onset of COVID-19 and government-issued "stay-at-home orders" may have driven these increases, the practice of TMH has remained steady since those restrictions have been lifted.

Describing TMH

The delivery of counseling services via the internet or other digital systems has had several titles over the years. While I primarily use "telemental health counseling (TMH)," other terms include *cyber counseling, e-therapy, internet-based counseling, distance counseling,* and *digital delivery of counseling services*. In a pre-COVID-19 study of 65 state licensure board websites, 42 different terms were utilized to explain the concept of TMH and counseling services, with 19 being more frequently cited. The terms *electronic counseling* or *electronic therapy* were the terms most often used among counseling and social work state licensing boards, whereas, among psychology state licensure boards, *telehealth* was the most prevalent term used (Ostrowski & Collins, 2016).

Different counseling specializations utilize different terms for TMH. The American Mental Health Counselor Association (AMHCA) uses *Technology Supported Counseling and Communications* (TSCC) in its 2023 Standards of Practice for Clinical Mental Health Counseling and its 2020 Code of Ethics. The American School Counselors Association (ASCA) refers to *virtual/distance school counseling* in its 2022 Code of Ethics. The National Career Development Association's (NCDA) 2015 Code of Ethics discusses *providing career services online* while also referring to the *use of technology and social media*. The National Board for Certified Counselors (NBCC) initially offered a policy regarding the *provision of distance professional services* (NBCC, 2016) and uses the terms *telemental health, social media, and technology* in its Code of Ethics (NBCC, 2023, p. 12).

Readers may note that the definitions used by some professional organizations do not contain the term *telemental health* (or TMH) when discussing distance services. One possible reason for not utilizing TMH within certain counseling specializations is that not all counseling professions involve mental health counseling. In fact, mental health counseling might not be included in the scope of practice for some specializations. Examples include career counseling, school counseling, and student affairs counseling. While these individuals may address the clients' and students' social and emotional needs, their scope of practice may or may not include mental health. Thus, while I use TMH throughout this book for consistency, I will be certain to note when the term may not be appropriate for some specializations.

National and international public health organizations often utilize terminology such as telehealth or telemedicine. Some organizations consider TMH included within telehealth/telemedicine, while others consider it a separate practice. SAMHSA (n.d.) utilizes "telemental health" in some contexts while using "telemedicine" or "telehealth" in other settings. The National Institute of Mental Health (NIMH, n.d.) refers to these services as "telemental health services" and recognizes that different terms, such as "telepsychology" and "telepsychiatry," may also be utilized. The Centers for Disease Control and Prevention (CDC, 2020) references "telemedicine" and "telehealth" but uses "telemental health" when specifically addressing mental health content. The World Health Organization (WHO, 2022) references "services via telehealth and telemedicine" and utilizes the term "digital health." Along with the International Telecommunication Union (ITU), WHO publishes standards for accessibility of telehealth services (WHO-ITU, 2022). Counselor educators and instructors recognize that different terminology for TMH may be used in other contexts.

Defining TMH

Definitions of TMH also vary. One of the earliest groups to define the concept of *web counseling* was the National Board for Certified Counselors (NBCC), which called it "the practice of professional counseling and information delivery that occurs when client(s) and counselor are in separate or remote locations and utilize electronic means to communicate over the Internet" (NBCC, 1997, p. 3). Professional organizations have created definitions that meet the needs of their profession. For example, when defining *Technology Supported Counseling and Communications* (TSCC), AMHCA's broach definition reads:

> B.6.a. CMHCs understand that the uses of TSCC in counseling may be considered to fall under the following categories: i.) The use of TSCC as the medium for counseling, also called "telehealth" or "distance counseling," includes but is not limited to the delivery of counseling by video call (e.g., internet, video chat), by voice (e.g., telephone), by synchronous text (e.g., chat or SMS), or by asynchronous text (e.g., email). ii.) The use of TSCC as an adjunct to counseling (i.e., for arranging, coordinating, or paying for counseling services), including the use of payment processing services that are integrated with TSCC (e.g., PayPal, Stripe, Zelle) for receipt of payment for counseling services. iii.). The use of online "cloud-based" services for the storage of counseling records. iv.) Marketing, educational

> forums, and other TSCC to include blogs, webpages, chatroom, etc. (AMHCA, 2020, p. 6)

In this AMHCA definition, TSCC includes providing counseling services via technology as well as technological communication, record keeping, and billing accompanying those services.

Federal agencies use other definitions of telehealth and telemedicine. The Health Resources and Services Administration (HRSA) states that "telehealth is defined as the use of electronic information and telecommunication technologies to support long-distance clinical health care, patient and professional health-related education, health administration, and public health" (HRSA, 2022, para. 1). Since the provision of telehealth services is often a component of insurance billing and medical payment, many organizations utilize the Medicaid definition of telehealth:

> Telehealth (or Telemonitoring) is the use of telecommunications and information technology to provide access to health assessment, diagnosis, intervention, consultation, supervision and information across distance. ... Telehealth includes such technologies as telephones, facsimile machines, electronic mail systems, and remote patient monitoring devices, which are used to collect and transmit patient data for monitoring and interpretation. (Center for Medicaid & Medicare Services, n.d., para. 13-14).

According to the Center for Connected Health Policy (CCHP), a program of the Public Health Institute, there is no single definition of telehealth, and definitions vary by state jurisdictions and settings. Again, counselor educators and instructors recognize that definitions of TMH may vary based on context and setting.

Prior TMH Knowledge

This book is not intended to provide instructors with initial training in TMH practice but to support the implementation of TMH concepts into counselor education and training. As addressed in the preface, this book assumes a baseline knowledge of TMH practice. This book will regularly utilize terms that are well-known in TMH practice settings but may not be familiar to all readers. The glossary at the end of this book is designed to define these terms, which will be denoted in bold as they appear and support the reader as they progress. Supplemental information may be needed to instruct with confidence and competence on issues of TMH. Before turning to this book, instructors who do not already have a baseline knowledge of TMH are encouraged to obtain this knowledge via training, reading, and practice.

Training

Professional development training programs in TMH have existed for many years. The American Counseling Association (ACA), in conjunction with Counseling Outfitters and Ready Minds, published the book *Distance Counseling: Expanding the Counselor's Reach and Impact* in 2007, indicating the early acceptance of TMH training within the profession (Malone et al., 2007). The Center for Credentialing and Education offers the Board Certified Telemental Health Provider (BC-TMH) credential (CCE, 2024). Originating as the Distance Counseling Credential (DCC), CCE transitioned to the BC-TMH in 2018. Other training and certificate programs in TMH are offered by well-regarded institutions such as the Zur Institute, PESI, and the American Telemedicine Association (ATA). These training programs vary in length, time, content, and cost (Robertson, 2021). There are free training programs available as well. The U.S. Department of Health and Human Services offers free telehealth training resources for providers (2024). However, there is no standard of TMH training, and no universal criteria have been established for TMH competence. Earlier research has unfortunately demonstrated a sense of confidence among practitioners utilizing TMH despite having limited, unsatisfactory, or no prior training (Baird et al., 2018; Cipoletta & Mocellin, 2018; Perle et al., 2012; Robertson & Lowell, 2021; Simms et al., 2011).

Training is not only recommended but an ethical imperative that is included within the ethical codes of organizations such as the ACA (2014), ASCA (2022), AMHCA (2020), and NCDA (2024), as well as others. For example, the ACA Code of Ethics addresses training in its discussion of counselor competence (Section C.2.a) and new specialty areas of practice (Section C.2.b; ACA, 2014). These codes indicate that counselors only engage in new areas of practice for which they received "education, training, and supervised experience" (ACA, 2014, p. 8). Section H.1.a specifies that "counselors who engage in the use of distance counseling, technology, and/or social media develop knowledge and skills regarding related technical, ethical, and legal considerations (e.g., special certifications, additional course work)" (ACA, 2014, p. 16). Similar standards are reflected within other professional organizations' ethical codes, and counselor educators should review those codes to identify the related provisions within their counseling specialization.

Reading

Counselor educators and instructors (henceforth "instructors") can pursue training programs, such as the BC-TMH mentioned above, or they may expand their knowledge through professional literature. A common misconception is that TMH is a "new" professional trend. TMH saw tremendous increases during and following the COVID-19 pandemic, yet the use of technology to provide counseling services has been in place for decades (Hornblow, 1986). As such, professional literature on TMH also spans decades.

Professional academic journals in counseling, psychology, social work, and other helping professions are good starting points for examining professional literature. When examining the literature, keep in mind that search terms may vary based on the multitude of titles used to describe and define TMH. More recently, targeted professional journals, such as the *Journal of Technology in Counselor Education and Supervision (JTCES),* published by the Western Association of Counselor Educators and Supervisors (WACES), focus exclusively on the use of technology in counselor education. Other specialized journals, such as the *Journal of Telemedicine and Telecare* and *Telehealth and Medicine Today,* focus on technology in delivering medical and mental health services. Following the onset of COVID-19, several professional journals dedicated special issues to COVID-19 interventions, including TMH.

Professional books on the practice of TMH continue to emerge. While individual research on TMH is useful, some instructors may seek a more comprehensive view of TMH through a book, as opposed to journal articles. While I completed the Distance Certified Counselor training in 2016 and additional training when transitioning to the BC-TMH in 2018, the books listed at the end of this chapter were particularly helpful in expanding my knowledge of TMH. I have also included some newer resources, as well as the book I authored in 2020 on TMH and distance counseling. Instructors are encouraged to seek updated resources and materials to remain current on TMH practice issues.

Practice

Instructors who are practicing counseling can expand their TMH skills by practicing via TMH modalities. As indicated above, counseling professional codes indicate that we gain competence through training and supervised practice. The 2024 Council for Accreditation of Counseling and Related Educational Programs (CACREP) standards include "ongoing counseling practice" (Standard 1.Z.3.c) as a faculty indicator of professional activities, scholarly activities, and service to the profession (CACREP, 2023). Thus, CACREP supports instructor engagement in ongoing counseling practice. Instructors who engage in counseling can seek supervision in TMH practice to expand their skills and comfort in providing TMH training to counselors-in-training (CITs).

Conclusion

Telemental health has become firmly embedded in the practice of professional counseling. Counselor educators and instructors are charged with educating the next generation of professional counselors to utilize TMH ethically and effectively with their clients and students. Instructors must understand the various descriptions and definitions of TMH and recognize that it is not a novel practice. Those without prior training can increase their knowledge in TMH via professional training, reading, and counseling practice.

Suggested Reading

Gilbertson, J. (2020). *Telemental health: The essential guide to providing successful online therapy.* PESI Publishing & Media.

Goss, S., Anthony, K., Stretch, L. S., Nagel, D. M. (2016). *Technology in mental health: Applications in practice, supervision, and training.* Charles C. Thomas.

Lutxon, D. D., Nelson, E., & Maheu, M. M. (2023). A practitioner's guide to telemental health: *How to conduct legal, ethical, and evidence-based telepractice* (2nd ed.). American Psychological Association.

Malone, J. F., Miller, R. K., & Walz, G. R. (Eds.). (2007). *Distance counseling: Expanding the counselor's reach and impact.* Counseling Outfitters, LLC.

Matheu, M. M. (2017). *Career paths in telemental health.* Springer.

Myers, K., & Turvey, C. (2012). *Telemental health: Clinical, technical, and administrative foundations for evidence-based practice.* Elsevier.

Robertson, H. C. (2021). *Telemental health and distance counseling: A counselor's guide to decisions, resources, and practice.* Springer Publishing Company.

Suggested Readings

[illegible] (2016). [illegible]

[illegible]

[illegible]

[illegible]

2

Teaching Telemental Health Practice

Before the pandemic, there was an ongoing debate about how mental health professionals should be trained in telemental health (TMH). Some felt that TMH training should be embedded into foundational graduate curricula. The fields of psychology and psychiatry strongly advocated for TMH training within the curriculum (Alicata et al., 2016; Glover et al., 2013; Hilty et al., 2015; Hoffman & Kane, 2013; Pullen et al., 2013; Sunderji et al., 2014). Others felt TMH training should be a post-training specialization (Anthony, 2015), following **face-to-face** (F2F) training in counseling. Psychology and psychiatry led early efforts to embed TMH into practice (Colbow, 2013), recognizing that TMH could increase access to much-needed psychological and psychiatric services. Some counselor educators have embraced TMH within master's level training, including TMH in content areas such as counseling skills (Trepal et al., 2007), group dynamics (Kozlowski & Holmes, 2017), and fieldwork (Haberstroh et al., 2008).

The U.S. Department of Health and Human Services (HHS) announced in March 2020 that it would waive **Health Insurance Portability and Accountability Act (HIPAA)** violations for practitioners during the pandemic (U.S. Department of Health and Human Services, 2020). This concession was designed to support the TMH continuum of care for those needing mental health and medical services; however, it may have inadvertently diverted practitioners from engaging in formal training. Professional development programs and TMH access continued to grow during the pandemic. PESI offered a free two-day, pre-recorded webinar to educate practitioners on the ethical practice of TMH. The online videoconference company Zoom offered free, unrestricted time when using their platform to support people in staying connected. Clinicians did whatever they could to continue practicing during this time, but TMH training may have been secondary to effectively engaging clients and students in counseling.

In a pre-COVID-19 study, 74 counselor educators were surveyed on how they taught TMH content within their counseling curriculum. Options included: not intentionally infused into their curriculum (26%), based on instructor preference (26%), intentionally infused into their curriculum (15%), offered as stand-alone elective on TMH (5%), and required as stand-alone class on TMH (1%; Robertson & Lowell, 2021). If that same study were administered today, many counselor educators would likely respond that they are trying to intentionally infuse TMH content into their curriculum. This book aims to support instructors in their efforts to infuse TMH content into an already crowded CACREP curriculum.

CACREP Lens

The Council for Accreditation of Counseling and Related Educational Programs (CACREP) exemplifies the profession's highest standard of counselor education. While other accreditation organizations exist, CACREP's 40-year history, national and international scope, and recognition from state and federal organizations as the standard for counselor training positions CACREP as a national model for counselor education programs. As such, this book uses a CACREP lens as the framework for providing TMH instructional information in relation to the core curriculum and specialization areas. The hope is that instructors may discover ways to weave TMH content into some of these areas without having to add an additional class in TMH to an already robust curriculum. While the CACREP standards have been included as I discuss each strategy, it may be helpful for the reader to have them available as a reference throughout their reading.

Prior versions of CACREP standards, specifically the 2009 and 2016 standards, do not mention the prospect of providing counseling via technology (CACREP, 2009; 2015), despite the National Board for Certified

Counselors (NBCC) publishing *Ethical Standards for Web-based Counseling* in 1997 (NBCC, 1997). The Center for Credentialing and Education (CCE) began providing Distance Counselor Certification (DCC) in conjunction with Ready Minds in 2004 (Shafer & Clawson, 2007). Despite these long-running developments within the profession, CACREP does not yet require counselor education programs to provide instruction in TMH.

There was no mention of technology, distance counseling, or digital delivery in the 2009 CACREP standards. The word "technology" only began to emerge in the 2016 CACREP standards, specifically, Standards 2.F.1 (Professional Orientation), 2.F.4 (Career Development), and the specialization curriculum standard 5.B.3 (Career Counseling) all mention technology (CACREP, 2015). Concerning career development, "technology" primarily referred to obtaining career information online, as opposed to providing counseling via technology. Beyond these three mentions of technology, no other references to "technology" or "digital delivery" are mentioned in the 2009 and 2016 standards.

The use of "technology" and "digital delivery" is addressed more frequently in the 2024 standards, but CACREP fails to require direct instruction in TMH. Standard 3.D.5 (Professional Orientation) requires that programs provide instruction on the "application of technology related to counseling" and uses the phrase "across service delivery modalities" at least twice (CACREP, 2023, p. 14). CACREP's directive to provide instruction on counseling across delivery modalities and on the application of technology to counseling signifies that counselor education programs should provide instruction to counselors-in-training (CITs) in both F2F and TMH modalities. While these cues are not explicit, they acknowledge the infusion of technology into the profession and the emergence of multiple counseling **modalities**. Throughout the book, I specifically cite CACREP standards and strategies to support the instruction of TMH in the core curriculum or specialized content areas.

Teaching Framework

CACREP's use of the phrase "across service delivery modalities" references the provision of counseling services. Instructors also provide training across delivery modalities. The pandemic changed many higher education institutions. Universities that operated primarily in an on-campus modality implemented significant changes to instructional methods. Many counselor education programs traditionally taught on campus had to quickly pivot to online modalities (Coker et al., 2021). Some state education departments provided concessions for online education and online supervision (e.g., New York Department of Education, 2020). Programs used different strategies to train counselors, such as technological software, to enhance counseling instruction (Chen et al., 2021). Much of the research from this period focuses on how education programs transitioned to online teaching and the mechanisms used to make that transition. Less research has been focused on how these education programs train students to use technology in TMH practice.

Today, instruction for CITs occurs via multiple modalities, including on-campus classrooms (sometimes called "bricks and mortar" or "on-ground" settings), virtual **synchronous** classrooms, virtual **asynchronous** classes, as well as hybrid and residential models that combine these modalities. TMH training for CITs must reflect the technological diversity with which it is delivered in the classroom.

On-Campus Classroom Instruction

Instructors who teach on campus have ample opportunity to teach and assess F2F counseling skills but will need access to additional technologies to adequately train and assess TMH skills. Lectures and didactic instruction can be delivered through traditional classroom methods, yet the practice and modeling of TMH will require supplemental technology. Universities may have access to technologies such as a **learning management system** (LMS) (e.g., Canvas, Blackboard, Google Classroom) or **videoconferencing** tools (e.g., WebEx, Teams, Zoom) that may not be available in agencies or smaller professional development training settings. Conversely, training offered through agencies or private practices may utilize **turnkey** or proprietary software (e.g., Simple Practice, TheraNest) unavailable to academic institutions. CITs will need access to **platforms** that allow them to learn, view, and demonstrate skills in video conferencing, phone, message, and email counseling. Using secure and **encrypted** technology, these platforms should allow them to practice their skills with mock clients or peers. The capacity to record, store, save, and transmit secure videos of students' mock counseling sessions is helpful. Yet, institutions need secure, **multifactor authentication** devices to store, submit, or send these recordings. Alternatively, instructors can utilize real-time observations via technology or view recorded videos with CITs in a shared location.

Online Synchronous Classroom Instruction

Instructors who teach in online synchronous settings can train and assess students in TMH, specifically in synchronous TMH counseling.

Lectures and didactic instruction can be delivered via synchronous instruction methods. Videoconferencing tools used to provide synchronous instruction, such as WebEx, Teams, and/or Zoom, may also be utilized to practice TMH skills, assuming they are secure and encrypted. Often, these tools provide options for video conferencing and chat, two modalities regularly utilized in TMH. In addition, the video component can be turned off to simulate telephone counseling while maintaining a secure connection without having students use personal mobile phones. Video and audio functionality can be turned off/muted to simulate **chat**-only sessions. Online synchronous instructional formats present a perfect opportunity to discuss and model online counseling skills. Instructors can model TMH skills in real-time during synchronous classes with volunteer students as mock clients. For effect, instructors can advise all other students to mute themselves and turn off their cameras while "pinning" the instructor and volunteer video to the screen, thus simulating the observation of a two-person TMH session. In addition, students can pair off into **breakout rooms** to conduct mock counseling sessions, where they can practice TMH skills; the instructor can drop in to observe sessions while muted and with their camera off for minimal distraction. While the online synchronous class is not a counseling group, it provides many tools and opportunities to simulate virtual group counseling. As discussed above, the capacity to record, store, save, and transmit secure videos or engage in real-time observation is helpful.

Online Asynchronous Classroom Instruction

Teaching TMH in purely an online asynchronous modality can present some challenges, particularly without the opportunity for real-time observation. For lecture and didactic instruction, instructors can post mock video and audio recordings or chat transcripts of TMH sessions to model ethical and effective TMH practice. To assess students' TMH skills, video and audio recordings of sessions should be submitted by students in alignment with the security and encryption features discussed above. Since the option for real-time observations or viewing recorded videos in a shared location is not an option in asynchronous settings, the capacity to record, store, save, and transmit secure videos of their counseling sessions is essential. Many online asynchronous programs utilize a residency or hybrid component; in this case, educators can utilize on-campus meetings or online synchronous instruction to provide training in the TMH practice.

Email Counseling

This brings me to the challenge of training students in email counseling, regardless of classroom setting. Email counseling is an asynchronous modality for TMH counseling utilized by some practitioners. In a TMH setting, counselors who use email counseling should utilize secure, encrypted email, using the address for client communication only. When training CITs in email counseling, instructors should use caution when students utilize their school or personal email, which could create a permanent record that can be accessed long after the class ends. Even though instructors often use "mock" clients during training, these mock clients may include peer students who share low-level personal concerns that are nonetheless confidential. Instructors need to utilize the same caution in disposing of these mock email transcripts as they would with actual client records, and all parties should understand that email leaves a **digital footprint**. An alternative to using actual email would be to use a word processing document to record the written dialogue, simulating back-and-forth email communication. This document would be sent back and forth between mock clients and counselors via a secure platform such as an LMS. Like recordings, the document needs to be appropriately disposed of after the course's conclusion.

Counselor-in-Training (CIT) Audience

Instructors come from various walks of life and hold different positions within the field. Some instructors hold positions as counselor education faculty at institutions of higher education. These positions include full-time, adjunct, clinical, teaching, tenure-track, and/or tenured faculty. We often think of counselor educators training master's or doctoral-level students in graduate counseling programs. Faculty may also teach associates, bachelor's, or continuing education students in courses leading to a different degree, such as a bachelor's in human services, or certification, such as a credential in addictions or peer counseling. Students in counselor education doctoral programs may be practicing instructors. Other instructors are not affiliated with institutions of higher education but instead work as professional trainers. Individual service agencies or large organizations may employ trainers focused on professional development. Still, other instructors may be practicing clinicians or supervisors charged with training other practitioners. Regardless of the setting or position, instructors (including counselor educators, faculty, trainers, and supervisors) who train counselors may be responsible for TMH training. Instructors often have experience in their area of instruction. Counselor educators have experience as professional counselors and may be required to hold a counseling license or certification to teach. However, depending on the area and setting in which they practiced, they may or may not have experience with TMH. As emphasized in Chapter 1, they need to have a foundational understanding of TMH before training others.

CITs, like instructors, come from various walks of life. This book uses a CACREP lens to create a teaching framework best aligned with master's training. However, as discussed above, CITs may be students at any educational level or professional counselors receiving additional training and continuing education. Like instructors, CITs may have extensive or limited experience with TMH. Many people desire to become professional counselors because they have benefited from professional counseling. Yet, their own personal counseling experience may not have included TMH either. In March 2020, during the onset of the COVID-19 pandemic, as we transitioned to online instruction and TMH practice, I remember some of my students resisting the transition to TMH. Their thought of seeing clients over a computer screen was not in their vision of counseling and not within their comfort zone. Fast-forward to March 2024, when most of my students who elected to share their own personal counseling experiences indicated that those occurred via TMH. CITs come to training with varying degrees of TMH comfort. Our goal is to meet them where they are and engage them in learning.

Understanding Andragogy

Counselor training typically occurs with adults. Whether providing instruction in a master's level CACREP program, bachelor's level instruction, or continuing education certification, the CITs are typically out of high school and often have completed a minimum of a bachelor's degree. Most would be classified as adults or young adults, yet CITs often include career changers and older adults transitioning to a new career. Unfortunately, many teaching and training approaches utilize pedagogy, the lens of instructing children and adolescents. How is teaching and training adults different from teaching and training children? More specifically, how do we most effectively teach TMH to adult CITs? Since most counselor training programs are graduate programs aimed at adult learners, Malcolm Knowles's concept of **andragogy** can be utilized for TMH instruction. Defined as "the art and science of helping adults learn," andragogy focuses on providing strategies to engage adult learners, as opposed to pedagogy aimed at children and adolescents (Knowles, 1975).

Andragogy embraces the needs of adult learners through four primary principles. The first is that learning should be self-directed. In general, graduate work is often driven by self-directed personal motivation, as opposed to legal mandate or parental pressure. This concept of self-direction is easily adapted to master's and doctoral-level training programs motivated by the individual's personal goals. Concerning TMH training, instructors should seek opportunities to provide self-directed learning when possible.

The second component of andragogy suggests that adult learners draw from their experiences when they approach learning, as suggested in my earlier commentary on students' familiarity and comfort with TMH. Instructors should seek opportunities to engage students' TMH experience in their learning while also providing practice TMH experiences for them to assess and evaluate. Providing ample practice with TMH during their training expands their lived experience with TMH, even in mock settings, and supports their learning.

The third principle states that adult learning occurs when there is a need for information. With the rapid increase of TMH practice, instructors can help CITs recognize the need to develop ethical and effective practice skills. More often, when CITs approach their fieldwork experiences, they will be challenged to engage in TMH practice. Those who have not had TMH training and practice throughout their education should not be learning these skills for the first time with actual clients and students in their fieldwork. Thus, the need to learn TMH concepts must be addressed before they meet with the public.

Finally, Knowles posits that adult learners prefer immediate learning application (Knowles, 1975). Regarding TMH training, instructors should provide timely opportunities for CITs to practice their acquired TMH skills and opportunities to use TMH in different modalities and settings, such as video, phone, chat, and email. Another component of immediate application is timely feedback. It is essential that CITs receive timely feedback on their TMH learning and have opportunities to correct any deficits and improve their practice.

This book will provide instructors with critical content, case studies, and lessons on the instruction of TMH, referencing adult learning while seeking to infuse andragogical concepts. By doing so, I hope the instruction you provide to CITs will be impactful, relevant, and sustained as they continue from the classroom into their TMH practice.

Foundational Counseling Curriculum

3

Professional Counseling Orientation and Ethical Practice

Ethics and professional identity are the foundation of professional counseling. These concepts shape our practice and service to clients and students alike. For those teaching in CACREP programs, Standard 3.E.5 (application of technology related to counseling) requires that instructors provide instruction on the "application of technology related to counseling" (CACREP, 2023, p. 14). The word "application" has been updated from the 2016 Standard 2.F.1.j, requiring instruction on "technology's impact on the counseling profession." The 2024 standard recognizes that technology will be applied to professional counseling, yet determining and defining how technology will be applied is at the discretion of the individual counseling program. Section 3.E uses the phrase "across service delivery modalities" at least twice (CACREP, 2023, p. 14), recognizing that counseling will be delivered across multiple modalities, including face-to-face (F2F) and TMH (telemental health). Once again, CACREP encourages programs to introduce the application of technology and counseling across multiple modalities but does not direct programs to provide specific TMH instruction.

Key Concepts

CACREP Standards

There are several key concepts that instructors will want to address as they introduce TMH to counselors-in-training (CITs) in the context of Section 3.A Professional Counseling Orientation and Ethical Practice. Since many programs utilize CACREP objectives in their teaching, Table 3.1 suggests how TMH content can be directly connected to specific standards. If these concepts are unfamiliar to the instructor, they should review the training and reading materials suggested in Chapter 1.

Table 3.1

CACREP Section 3.A (Professional Counseling Orientation and Ethical Practice) and Suggested TMH Content

CACREP Standards (2024)	Suggested TMH Content
3.A. History and philosophy of the counseling profession and its specialized practice areas.	History of the emergence of TMH (Breen & Matusitz, 2010; Hornblow, 1986).
3.A.2. The multiple professional roles and functions of counselors across specialized practice areas.	Exploration of how TMH and distance counseling are used among various specializations, such as school counseling and career counseling (Robertson, 2021).
3.A.3. Counselors' roles, responsibilities, and relationships as members of specialized practice and interprofessional teams, including (a) collaboration and consultation, (b) community outreach, and (c) emergency response management.	Use of technology and TMH in emergency and crisis services (e.g., phone/text hotlines) (Predmore et al., 2017).
3.A.4. The role and process of the professional counselor advocating on behalf of and with individuals receiving counseling services to address systemic, institutional, architectural, attitudinal, disability, and social barriers that impede access, equity, and success.	The use of TMH in expanding access to rural and specialized communities compounded with barriers in access to TMH treatment based on education, socioeconomic status (SES), and geographic region (see Chapter 4).

CACREP Standards (2024)	Suggested TMH Content
3.A.5. The role and process of the professional counselor advocating on behalf of the profession.	Discussion on the **Counseling Compact** (2024) and the advocacy efforts for TMH treatment across states.
3.A.6. Professional counseling organizations, including membership benefits, activities, services to members, and current issues.	Currently, no ACA division is focused on TMH, but some professional journals and interest groups within some organizations exist (e.g., ACA Connect Interest Networks in Counseling & Technology, Distance Learning, and Artificial Intelligence).
3.A.7. Professional counseling credentialing across service delivery modalities, including certification, licensure, and accreditation practices and standards for all specialized practice areas.	Discussion of TMH credentialing, including the Board Certified TeleMental Health Provider (BC-TMH). Exploration of state licensure guidelines pertaining to TMH practice (Epstein, Becker, & Green, 2024).
3.A.8. Legislation, regulatory processes, and government/public policy relevant to and impact on service delivery of professional counseling across service delivery modalities and specialized practice areas.	Continued discussion on Counseling Compact and state laws/licensing (Standards 3.A.5 and 3.A.7).
3.A.9. Current labor market information and occupational outlook relevant to opportunities for practice within the counseling profession.	Capacity for TMH to address counselor **Health Professional Shortage Areas** (HPSA; HRSA, 2019).
3.A.10. Ethical standards of professional counseling organizations and credentialing bodies, and applications of ethical and legal considerations in professional counseling across service delivery modalities and specialized practice areas.	A significant area of discussion (see further content in this chapter).
3.A.11. Self-care, self-awareness, and self-evaluation strategies for ethical and effective practice.	Propensity for TMH practice to blur professional work/life balance issues (e.g., in-home practice, COVID-19).
3.A.12. The purpose of and roles within counseling supervision in the profession.	Applies to e-supervision practices (see Chapter 19 for references).

Professional Ethics

Ethical practice is the foundation of professional counseling, and TMH counseling is no different. Instructors have a critical responsibility to advise CITs on the ethical and professional challenges of practicing via technology. As discussed in Chapter 1, previous research and the COVID-19 pandemic demonstrate that some counselors have engaged in TMH practice with little to no training and may risk violating ethical components that TMH practice demands. While a full review of ethical concepts is covered in the TMH trainings and readings suggested in Chapter 1, instructors and CITs should critically examine ethical codes and how these principles impact TMH.

The American Counseling Association Code of Ethics provides a separate section on TMH practice entitled "Section H: Distance Counseling, Technology, and Social Media" (ACA, 2014). The entirety of this code can be applied to TMH practice. Professional counselors (and CITs) are responsible for knowing and adhering to the complete document, not just Section H, even if they practice solely via TMH. Table 3.2 highlights key ethical concepts instructors should reinforce during TMH training related to the ACA Code of Ethics. Although not inclusive of all areas, instructors should cross-reference the sections outlined in Table 3.2 with the specific wording of the ethical code, then apply the TMH ethical construct discussed to their lesson. Again, if these concepts are unfamiliar, Chapter 1 provides training and reading materials to assist in gaining familiarity with these concepts.

Table 3.2

ACA Code of Ethics Standards and Suggested TMH Content

ACA Code of Ethics (2014)	Suggested Emphasis for TMH Ethics
Section A: The Counseling Relationship.	A.1.b., Digital storage of records; A.2., F2F & TMH informed consent differences (see additional information to follow); A.5.e., Personal virtual relationships prohibited; A.7., Advocacy for TMH access; A.9., Group Work (see Chapter 8); A.11., Termination via TMH; A.12., Abandonment via TMH.

ACA Code of Ethics (2014)	Suggested Emphasis for TMH Ethics
Section B: Confidentiality and Privacy.	B.1.b., Challenges of privacy in TMH sessions; B.1.c., Risks to confidentiality in TMH sessions; B.2.a., Challenges with duty to warn via TMH; B.4., TMH group work and families (see Chapters 8 & 16); B.6., Digital storage and transmission of records and documentation. Section B has significant relevance to TMH, specifically regarding encryption, privacy, security, HIPAA, and **Business Associate Agreements** (BAA) (see specifics in Section H).
Section C: Professional Responsibility.	C.2.a., Boundaries of competence in using TMH; C.2.b., New areas of practice – TMH; C.2.f., Continuing education in TMH; C.2.g., TMH blurring boundaries between work/home/wellness – monitor for impairment; C.4.b., Accurate representation of TMH credentials; C.5., Nondiscrimination – recognition that TMH creates both opportunities and obstacles for some clients (Chapter 4), C.6.b., Discussion of third-party software and data security; C.7., Application to TMH treatment modalities
Section D: Relationship with Other Professionals.	D.1., Different employers and professions may utilize TMH differently and follow different ethical codes or practice standards; D.2., Following appropriate security and informed consent measures if providing TMH consultation.
Section E: Evaluation, Assessment, and Interpretation.	See Chapter 9.
Section F: Supervision, Training, and Teaching.	See Chapters 19 and 20.
Section G: Research and Publication.	See Chapter 10.

ACA Code of Ethics (2014)	Suggested Emphasis for TMH Ethics
Section H: Distance Counseling, Technology, and Social Media.	Full exploration and discussion of Section H is required in TMH training; all sections must be understood and adhered to for ethical TMH practice. Additional information on informed consent is included below.
Section I: Resolving Ethical Issues.	I.1., State laws on TMH practice; I.2., Challenges of identifying and reporting violations among practitioners.

The National Board for Certified Counselors (NBCC) Code of Ethics (2023) focuses 23 of their 114 standards on "Telemental Health, Social Media, and Technology" (items 91–114). In many ways, these items align with Section H of the ACA Code of Ethics. NBCC ethical standards tend to be more individualized and detailed, particularly concerning screening (item 99) and intake (item 100). Conversely, ACA codes often encompass several NBCC items within one standard. One area specifically mentioned within ACA's Section H that is not included in the NBCC code is multicultural and disability considerations (H.5.d).

Respectively, NBCC codes include content on TMH services with minors (item 104) and the use of **privacy settings** in **social media** (item 110), which is not explicitly mentioned in the ACA Code. Table 3.3 outlines the parallels between the two codes. In this book, Appendix A includes the complete Section H (Distance Counseling) of the ACA Code of Ethics (2014) and Telemental Health, Social Media, and Technology (items 91-114) from the NBCC Code of Ethics (2023), which is a helpful reference to the table below.

Table 3.3

Alignment between NBCC (2023) and ACA (2014) TMH Standards

NBCC Standards	ACA Standards
Item 91	H.1.a
Item 92	H.1.b
Item 93	H.1.b, H.2.d
Item 94	H.2.d
Item 95	H.5.a

NBCC Standards	ACA Standards
Item 96	H.4.b
Item 97	H.2.a, H.4.a
Item 98	H.2.c
Item 99	H.4.c
Item 100	H.4.c, H.4.d, H.4.e
Item 101	H.2.b
Item 102	H.2.a, H.5.b
Item 103	H.2.c
Item 104	N/A – TMH and minors
Item 105	H.2.a
Item 106	H.3
Item 107	H.6.b, H.6.c
Item 108	H.5.a
Item 109	H.2.a
Item 110	N/A – Social media privacy
Item 111	H.6.d
Item 112	H.6.a
Item 113	H.6.c
Item 114	H.4.b

Informed Consent

Informed consent documents outline critical information on the counseling relationship and signify client and student awareness and agreement to participate in counseling. When providing TMH training, instructors are encouraged to help CITs closely examine the various components of informed consent in both F2F and TMH counseling settings. This can be accomplished by comparing Standards A.2.a (Informed Consent), A.2.b (Types of Information Needed), and H.2.a (Informed Consent and Disclosure) in the ACA Code of Ethics (2014). Beyond the information required in all counseling informed consent documents (outlined in

Standards A.2.a and A.2.b), Standard H.2.a includes additional TMH elements, including but not limited to "distance counseling credentials, physical location of practice ... risks and benefits of engaging in distance counseling, technology, and/or social media ... possibility of technology failure ... anticipated response time ... [and] social media policies" (ACA, 2014, p. 18). Some of those risks and benefits include informing clients of the possibility of data breaches, the risk of using third-party software vendors, and the steps used to protect client identity and information.

Teaching Techniques

Instructors can introduce the issues of TMH ethical practice in a variety of ways. Below is a list of suggested strategies that might reinforce or supplement CITs' understanding of TMH and professional ethics. These strategies utilize the andragogical principles previously discussed in Chapter 2, including self-motivated learning, using prior experiences, recognizing a need for information, and immediately applying learning in real-world contexts (Knowles, 1975).

1. *State laws, and the ACA and NBCC Codes of Ethics*. Examine state laws, including the scope of counseling practice and specifications for TMH. Ask CITs to explore potential conflicts between TMH state laws and TMH ethical codes.
2. *Re-examine ethical cases from a TMH lens*. Ethical case studies from textbooks or other sources can be recrafted or reimagined from a TMH perspective for CITs to explore how ethical issues evolve when practiced in both F2F and TMH settings.
3. *TMH Case Studies*. Use or create TMH case studies focused on ethical issues.
4. *TMH Informed Consent*. Have CITs write one informed consent document for TMH practice and one for F2F practice. Explore variations in language and audience.
5. *Third-Party Software Security Analysis*. Select a third-party software utilized in TMH practice. These may include turnkey platforms or tools used to support TMH (such as videoconferencing). Have CITs examine the publicly available standards for encryption, security, data management, data storage, and HIPAA compliance.
6. *Business Associate Agreement (BAA)*. Request or examine a BAA from a third-party vendor. Have CITs examine how the agreement aligns with counseling laws and ethics.

7. *Duty to Warn and Emergency Contact.* Role-play the duty to warn using emergency contacts in TMH modalities, including video, phone, text, or email sessions. Have CITs discuss the steps needed to ethically approach these cases when establishing a TMH practice.
8. *Multistate Licensure.* Explore licensure requirements and scope of practice pertaining to TMH in multiple states of desired practice. Have CITs consider how the Counseling Compact could be both a support and challenge for ethical TMH practice and client safety.
9. *Prior Experiences with TMH.* CITs may have previously engaged in TMH counseling or been exposed to TMH through media and other sources. CITs can evaluate their prior experiences (via a journal or small group discussion) and the ethics of their experiences.
10. *TMH Practice Self-Care Plan.* Ask CITs to imagine they were operating a home-based TMH private practice. Have them develop a self-care plan to maintain their wellness and practice in such a space.

Sample Lesson: Role of Ethics in Telemental Health Delivery

John J. S. Harrichand, PhD, LPC-S, LMHC, NCC, ACS
University of Texas at San Antonio

Lesson Objectives

1) Educate Counselors-in-Training (CITs) on applicable TMH codes and policies.
2) Apply TMH laws, informed consent, client verification, and the distance counseling relationship via a case study.
3) Synthesize knowledge through critical discussions following the activity.

2024 CACREP Standards

Section 3.E (Counseling Practice and Relationships), Standards 3.E.5 (Application of technology related to counseling), 3.E.6 (Ethical and legal issues relevant to establishing and maintaining counseling relationships across service delivery modalities), and 3.E.7 (Culturally sustaining and responsive strategies for establishing and maintaining counseling relationships across service delivery modalities).

Materials and/or Technology Required

1) The ACA Code of Ethics (2014)
2) The National Board for Certified Counselors (NBCC) Code of Ethics (2023)
3) Case Example

Preparation Required

Access to ACA and NBCC Codes and the case study (digital and/or print).

Estimated Time Required for Lesson Delivery

The total time for this activity is approximately 60–90 minutes, depending on classroom size. Time modifications can be made based on instructor needs and/or depth of discussion. At least 20 minutes of discussion will be needed for this activity.

- 60–70 minutes to review and process the case study.
- 20–30 minutes for question-and-answer discussion.

Structure and Audience for Lesson

The lesson can be delivered synchronously online or in-person to graduate counseling students in any CACREP specialty area.

Lesson Content and Instructional Strategies

The ACA Code of Ethics (2014) provides counselors with best practices regarding ethical behavior and decision-making, allowing for professional relationships to develop focused on empowering diverse clients and communities to recognize and accomplish their goals. The ethical codes contain specific guidance for Distance Counseling, Technology, and Social Media under Section H of the Standards to assist counselors in "avoiding harm, determining appropriateness [for online counseling], and awareness of risk and/or liability" (Robertson, 2021, p. 44).

Counselors desirous of practicing TMH must receive training and demonstrate competence in using technology and applying clinical skills in a distance setting (Robertson, 2021; Robertson & Lowell, 2021). Section

H of the ACA Code of Ethics (2014) provides counselors, regardless of practice modality (i.e., in-person or online), with guidance in six areas:

1. Knowledge and Legal Considerations
2. Informed Consent and Security
3. Client Verification
4. Distance Counseling Relationship
5. Records and Web Maintenance
6. Social Media.

Similarly, the NBCC Code of Ethics (2023) provides 18 codes, numbered 91–108, under the Telemental Health, Social Media, and Technology section, guiding counselors engaged in TMH counseling. The 18 codes include encryption of all digital communication, screening potential clients for distance services, counseling a minor, emergency contacts, accessing client information via social media platforms, and time limitations for retaining records. Depending on the CIT's and/or the counselor's state of residence and counseling practice, it is their responsibility to know relevant laws and statutes governing their practice of TMH. They can obtain this information through their state's licensing or certification boards (Robertson, 2021).

Case Example

Rupa, a 28-year-old East Indian Hindu immigrant woman, is a recent counseling graduate from a CACREP-accredited program in south Texas who was hired at a rural mental health clinic in the same state. She is tasked with conducting both in-person and virtual counseling sessions with children and adults who are immigrants and refugees. Rupa is currently working toward earning her professional counselor license, which will allow her to practice independently. During her internship experience, she offered online counseling through the clinic connected to her department. Today, she was informed by the front desk staff that she would be meeting with a male refugee teenager from Central America who is a member of the LGBTQ+ community, followed by an older adult Muslim female immigrant from Africa, via distance counseling. Based on the information provided, specific to Rupa's two clients, use the prompts to address important TMH considerations.

1. Either in dyads/triads or groups, have students participate in a think-pair-share activity, identifying:
   a. What relevant ACA Section H codes apply? Why?
   b. What relevant NBCC codes apply? Why?
   c. What relevant state laws and codes apply, e.g., the Texas Behavioral Health Executive Council? Why?
2. Regarding Rupa's informed consent, what needs to be included? Why?
3. What are important confidentiality considerations for Rupa to note when meeting both clients? How might she address them in their session?
4. What suggestions do you have for helping Rupa verify her clients? How often should Rupa participate in client verification and why?
5. Role-play Activity:
   a. Pretend you are Rupa meeting with either the teenage LGBTQ+ client or the older female Muslim client; role-play with your peer about how you would initiate contact via distance counseling.
   b. Provide feedback to each other on strengths and areas for growth.

Assessment of Objectives

- What are some key things you have learned about TMH counseling from this activity?
- What if anything surprised you about TMH counseling?
- What are some potential challenges related to TMH counseling?
- How do you plan on incorporating information learned from this lesson into your future role as a counselor?

References

American Counseling Association. (2014). *2014 ACA code of ethics.* https://www.counseling.org/Resources/aca-code-of-ethics.pdf

Chandler, A. (2020, September 1). Making the 'new' normal: Five tips for providing teletherapy.

Counseling Today. https://ct.counseling.org/2020/09/making-the-new-normal-five-tips-for-providing-teletherapy/

National Board for Certified Counselors. (2023). *NBCC code of ethics*. https://www.nbcc.org/assets/Ethics/nbcccodeofethics.pdf

Robertson, H. C. (2021). *Telemental health and distance counseling: A counselor's guide to decisions, resources, and practice* (pp. 43–65). Springer.

Robertson, H. C., & Lowell, R. (2021). Counselor educator, supervisor, and practitioner perspectives on distance counseling and telemental health training and practice. *Journal of Counselor Preparation and Supervision, 14*(3), 1–32. https://digitalcommons.sacredheart.edu/jcps/vol14/iss3/3

Texas Behavioral Health Executive Council. (n.d.). *Statutes and rules*. https://www.bhec.texas.gov/statues-and-rules/index.html

Sample Lesson: Law, Ethics, and Credentialing: Attempting to Make Sense of Guidance When Utilizing Telemental Health as a Clinical Modality

Matthew R. Shupp, EdD, NCC, BC-TMH, ACS, LPC
Shippensburg University of Pennsylvania

Lesson Objectives

Students will:

1) Compare and contrast legal mandates, ethical codes, and credentialing standards when utilizing telemental health as a clinical modality.
2) Name and identify key legal mandates and ethical standards when utilizing telemental health as a clinical modality.
3) Examine strengths and limitations when using telemental health modalities when conducting clinical therapy.

CACREP Standards (2024)

Standards 3.A.7 (Professional counseling credentialing, including certification, licensure, and accreditation practices and standards for specialized practice areas), 3.A.8 (Legislation, regulatory processes, and government/public policy relevant to and impact on professional counseling and specialized practice areas), and 3.A.10 (Ethical standards of professional counseling organizations and credentialing bodies, and applications of ethical and legal considerations in professional counseling).

Materials and/or Technology Required

Instructor laptop and projector, internet/Wi-Fi access, student laptops and/or smartphones, access to the ACA Code of Ethics (2014), and access to an online digital platform such as Padlet (preferred), Kahoot, or Mentimeter.

Preparation Required

Create an access account in one of the digital platforms mentioned above so students can utilize the platform in real-time. Padlet will be used for this example.

Estimated Time Required for Lesson Delivery

1.5–2 hours.

Structure and Audience for Lesson

Ideally, this activity works best in graduate training programs where students can work together in small groups (approximately 3 students per group). If technology allows for synchronous virtual learning, the activity could be conducted in a virtual space.

Lesson Content and Instructional Strategies

This lesson would ideally occur after in-depth discussions on professional counseling credentialing, legal mandates, legislation, regulatory processes, and ethical standards to tie together the complexity and nuance associated with such weighty topics.

Have students break into groups of 2–3 students/group. Instructors could provide an overview of state regulations/laws or credentialing agencies as part of the initial setup. For this example, use the core professional values stated in the ACA Code of Ethics:

1. Enhancing human development throughout the life span
2. Honoring diversity and embracing a multicultural approach in support of the worth, dignity, potential, and uniqueness of people within their social and cultural contexts
3. Promoting social justice
4. Safeguarding the integrity of the counselor–client relationship, and
5. Practicing in a competent and ethical manner (ACA, 2014). The six ethical pillars of the profession should also be considered:
   a. *Autonomy*, or fostering the right to control the direction of one's life,
   b. *Nonmaleficence*, or avoiding actions that cause harm,
   c. *Beneficence*, or working for the good of the individual and society by promoting mental health and well-being,
   d. *Justice*, or treating individuals equitably and fostering fairness and equality,
   e. *Fidelity*, or honoring commitments and keeping promises, including fulfilling one's responsibilities of trust in professional relationships, and
   f. *Veracity*, or dealing truthfully with individuals with whom counselors come into professional contact (ACA, 2014).

Next, each group will be asked to choose and discuss a particular ethical standard from Section H (Distance Counseling, Technology, and Social Media) (ACA, 2014, pp. 17–18). Below are a few examples and prompts for discussion and consideration.

Example 1. Standard H.1.a, Knowledge and Competency (read aloud the description)

Q: What does "develop knowledge and skills" mean? Is there a minimum standard?

Example 2. Standard H.1.b, Laws and Statutes (read aloud the description)

Q: "May be subject to law and regulations of both...location and... place of residence." What does this look like in practice related to vacations, work trips, and so on?

Example 3. H.2.a, Informed Consent and Disclosure (read aloud the description)

Q: Do you include all of this information as part of your intake paperwork?

Example 4. H.2.d, Security (read aloud the description)

Q: What are best practices as it relates to encryption standards? Does this change if a counselor uses technology/internet services from an office versus their home?

Example 5. H.3, Client Verification (read aloud the description)

Q: For you, does "distance counseling" include phone sessions? What are the most appropriate steps to ensure the client's identity?

Example 6. H.4.a, Benefits and Limitations (read aloud the description)

Q: What happens if a client is in crisis? What protocols have been established?

Additional Prompts

- How would you identify if clients are of appropriate cognitive disposition to benefit from telemental health?
- What ethical reasonability do we have to provide telemental health services as a means of equity to accessible services?

Students should be given adequate time to discuss the question prompts and how they plan to provide their responses and rationale to the group. This exercise's aim is not just to move beyond basic recall of ethical standards but is also intended to train students to integrate and synthesize material into an organized format to aid their practical application of said standards.

Research indicates that co-created material, by elevating student voices and actively engaging in creating course content, often results in stronger retention of material (Katz, 2021). Padlet is a user-friendly platform that allows learners to collaborate online by posting content (e.g., text, images, links, documents, videos, and voice recordings) in real-time. Once given access to the particular Padlet (usually set up by the instructor), students work in groups to add/edit content and create rubrics, as well as access the material(s) long after the subject matter has been discussed.

Assessment of Objectives

Instructors create a rubric to assess student learning or review outcomes related to content on Padlet. Some examples of rubric standards could include Sophisticated (clearly organized, uses outside research), Acceptable (generally focused, mostly clear), Developing (somewhat unfocused or lacking depth but had coherence), Inadequate (at least one serious weakness, underdeveloped), and Unsatisfactory (incomplete, unorganized).

Additional Resources

Many free, basic online learning tools are available for student collaboration. Consider how you might alter this lesson by utilizing a different learning tool.

- Kahoot: https://kahoot.com/schools-u/
- Mentimeter: https://www.mentimeter.com/
- Padlet: https://padlet.com/

References

American Counseling Association. (2014). *ACA code of ethics.*

Center for Credentialing and Education, Inc. (n.d.). https://www.cce-global.org/

Pennsylvania Code and Bulletin (n.d.). *Chapter 49, State Board of Social Workers, Marriage and Family Therapists and Professional Counselors.* https://www.pacodeandbulletin.gov/

Council for Accreditation of Counseling and Related Educational Programs (CACREP; 2023). *2024 Standards.*

Katz, S. (2021). Co-creating with students: practical considerations and approaches. *Times Higher Education.* https://www.timeshighereducation.com/campus/cocreating-students-practical-considerations-and-approaches

National Board for Certified Counselors (NBCC). (2023). *Code of ethics.*

4

Social and Cultural Identities and Experiences

Multiculturalism has been defined as the fourth force in counseling (Pedersen, 1991), while social justice is argued to be the fifth (Ratts, 2009). Despite these early proclamations, there are continued calls to decolonize the profession and move toward counseling interventions that fully embrace multiculturalism and social justice in our counseling work (Singh et al., 2020). While telemental health (TMH) can create opportunities to diversify access to our profession, it can also create access barriers for marginalized populations. Counselors-in-training (CITs) will need to understand TMH opportunities and setbacks as they begin their practice.

Key Concepts

CACREP Standards

There are several key concepts that instructors will want to address as they introduce TMH in conjunction with social and cultural identities. Many programs utilize CACREP objectives in their teaching. Table 4.1 provides suggestions on how TMH content connects to CACREP standards. If these concepts are unfamiliar, the instructor is reminded to explore the training and reading materials suggested in Chapter 1.

Table 4.1

CACREP Section 3.B (Social and Cultural Identities and Experiences) and Suggested TMH Content

CACREP Standards (2024)	Suggested TMH Content
3.B.1. Theories and models of multicultural counseling, social justice, and advocacy.	Exploration of how multicultural theories and models can be adapted for and impacted by TMH delivery.
3.B.2. The influence of heritage, cultural identities, attitudes, values, beliefs, understandings, within-group differences, and acculturative experiences on individuals' worldviews.	Capacity for TMH to connect clients and preferred counselors from shared cultural identities, beliefs, and world views; different online communities for cultural groups.
3.B.3. The influence of heritage, cultural identities, attitudes, values, beliefs, understandings, within-group differences, and acculturative experiences on help-seeking and coping behaviors.	Exploring stigma of help-seeking among cultural communities, e.g., men (Masho & Alvanzo, 2010), African American (Avent Harris et al., 2020; Neely-Fairbanks et al., 2018), Asian (Han & Pong, 2015), and Latine cultures (Menendez et al., 2020).
3.B.4. The effects of historical events, multigenerational trauma, and current issues on diverse cultural groups in the U.S. and globally.	Mental health impact of historical events, multigenerational trauma, and current issues and need for mental health care for marginalized populations (F2F or TMH).
3.B.5. The effects of stereotypes, overt and covert discrimination, racism, power, oppression, privilege, marginalization, microaggressions, and violence on counselors and clients.	Mental health impact of stereotypes, overt and covert discrimination, racism, power, oppression, privilege, marginalization, microaggressions, and violence and the need for mental health care for marginalized populations (F2F or TMH).
3.B.6. The effects of various socio-cultural influences, including public policies, social movements, and cultural values, on mental and physical health and wellness.	Digital divide and infrastructure limitations of TMH (see later in this chapter).
3.B.7. Disproportional effects of poverty, income disparities, and health disparities toward people with marginalized identities.	Health Professional Shortage Areas (HPSA; HRSA, 2023); infrastructure barriers despite capacity for TMH to create access; demographic disparities.

CACREP Standards (2024)	Suggested TMH Content
3.B.8. Principles of independence, inclusion, choice and self-empowerment, and access to services within and outside the counseling relationship.	Capacity for TMH to create independence, inclusion, choice, self-empowerment, and access to services and specialists (e.g., telepsychiatry; gender-affirming care).
3.B.9. Strategies for identifying and eliminating barriers, prejudices, and processes of intentional and unintentional oppression and discrimination.	Counseling Compact; Infrastructure advocacy; capacity for TMH to improve access in rural communities and Medicare recipients (Mehrotra et al., 2017; Patel et al., 2020; Weiss et al., 2018), and people with disabilities (see Chapter 14).
3.B.10. Guidelines developed by professional counseling organizations related to social justice, advocacy, and working with individuals with diverse cultural identities.	Examining the Multicultural and Social Justice Counseling Competencies (MSJCC; Ratts et al., 2015) from technological privilege (see further content in this chapter).
3.B.11. The role of religion and spirituality in clients' and counselors' psychological functioning.	Capacity for TMH to connect clients and counselors from faith-based communities; Concerns surrounding qualifications of providers providing services that qualify as specific-spiritual counseling (F2F or TMH); Specific platforms or online searches targeting spiritual counseling.

Multicultural and Social Justice Counseling Competencies

The Multicultural and Social Justice Counseling Competencies (MSJCC) were adopted in 2015 by the ACA Governing Council (Ratts et al., 2015). While not directly aimed at TMH, the framework allows instructors and CITs to evaluate TMH practice from a multicultural and social justice lens. Competency I, Counselor Self-Awareness, begins with awareness of our own "social identities, social group statuses, power, privilege, oppression, strengths, limitations, assumptions, attitudes, values, beliefs, and biases" (p. 5). Competency II, Client Worldview, includes "curiosity for privileged and marginalized clients' history, worldview, cultural background, values, beliefs, biases, and experiences" (p. 6). Instructors are encouraged to challenge CITs to consider questions such as: What power, privilege, assumptions, attitudes, beliefs, and biases do I hold concerning technology, using technology, and having access to technology? What type of access, understanding, and limitations with technology do my clients and students have? How might these impact access to my TMH practice?

Competency III, Counseling Relationships, states that counselors "acknowledge that the counseling relationship may extend beyond the traditional office setting and into the community" (Ratts et al., 2015, p. 9), which reflects the practice of TMH services. Competency IV, Counseling Advocacy and Interventions, considers social and systemic inequities that reduce access, such as infrastructure and inequities in accessing technology. The MSJCC provides a framework to explore TMH power and privilege and to consider technological access and assumptions.

The Digital Divide

Telemental health requires counselors and clients to have access to technology. TMH can increase counseling access for various cultural groups, but that access is only possible for those with compatible technology. The **digital divide** creates significant disparities in the U.S. based on geographic regions and racial, socioeconomic, and educational differences. Instructors can help CITs recognize that equitable and effective TMH requires an awareness of the population they plan to serve and its access to technology. If the population does not have access to technology, CITs must explore other means of providing services.

Home **broadband** and **smartphones** are two types of technology typically needed to engage in TMH. Broadband allows faster streaming of video and other internet content, which is less likely to result in the lagging and slowing down of internet services. Smartphones enable many people to utilize TMH services without a laptop or personal computer. Access to both broadband and smartphones varies. In 2021, according to a Pew Research Center study, access to smartphones was almost equal among racial groups of White (85%), Black (83%), and Hispanic (85%) U.S. adults. Yet, in other areas, differences were stark. Among various age groups, only 61% of adults over 65 had access to a smartphone compared to 96% of those ages 18–29. Educational disparities indicated that only 75% of adults with a high school education had a smartphone compared to 93% of those with a college degree. Finally, from a socioeconomic perspective, 76% of those with an income of under $30,000/annually had a smartphone compared to 96% of those who earned $75,000/annually or more. Broadband disparities were even more significant in some categories. For example, 92% of households earning over $75,000/annually had broadband compared to 57% of those earning less than $30,000/annually. Among adults with a high school education, 59% had broadband, compared to 94% of those with a college degree (Perrin, 2021).

Teaching Techniques

Instructors and CITs can explore TMH applications through a lens of social and cultural identity and experience. Below is a list of suggested strategies that might reinforce or supplement CITs' understanding of TMH and multicultural competence. These strategies utilize the andragogical principles discussed in Chapter 2, including self-motivated learning, using prior experiences, recognizing a need for information, and immediately applying learning in real-world contexts (Knowles, 1975).

1. *Multicultural Counseling Theories and TMH.* CITs learn several approaches to counseling diverse populations. Have CITs explore how utilizing TMH may impact multicultural counseling interventions, if at all.
2. *Cultural Counselor Characteristics.* Brainstorm cultural characteristics that clients/students might seek in counselors. Consider all areas of culture and identity, including gender, race, language, sexual orientation, disability, religion, geographic region, military status, and socioeconomic status. Have CITs come up with as many characteristics as possible and discuss how or why a client might find these shared characteristics desirable in a counselor.
3. *Finding Diverse Counselors Online.* Using the list that CITs created in suggestion #2, have CITs use the internet to identify counselors that meet some of the desired characteristics. How easy would it be for clients to find these counselors? What online tools did CITs use? How confident are they in the counselor's ability to be culturally affirming in the desired area?
4. *Research Counseling Affinity Groups.* Have CITs research counseling affinity groups. Examples include services aimed at religious beliefs, LGBTQ+, and others. What information can they find on the practice? What training or criteria do the counselors in this practice have in relation to the affinity group? How confident are CITs that the counselor will be ethical and affirming? What might be the pros/cons or risks/benefits of these groups?
5. *Explore Health Professional Shortage Areas* (HPSA). Using the U.S. Department of Health Resources and Services Administration website (n.d., https://data.hrsa.gov/tools/shortage-area), have

CITs research HPSAs in their state for mental health providers. Have CITs share what they learn/discover about access to mental health care in their region or other areas they might practice in the future. What is the demographic background of people in that region? How might that impact their access to mental health care?

6. *Counseling Compact.* Have CITs explore which states have signed the Counseling Compact. How will the compact increase or hinder access to care for marginalized communities? How might the compact impact counseling practices? https://counselingcompact.org/
7. *Cross-reference HPSA and Counseling Compact.* Have CITs cross-reference HPSAs with states that have signed the Compact. How will the Compact increase or hinder access to care for mental health HPSA communities? What about those not in the Compact?
8. *Technology Requirements for TMH Practice.* Have CITs explore their state licensing TMH requirements. Do state guidelines specify the provider's bandwidth or encryption level requirements? If so, how would that impact your TMH practice and client access?
9. *Research State Bandwidth.* Use the U.S. Census's "Digital Equity Act Population Viewer" to examine internet access in different states. For a selected state, explore the percentage of broadband-covered households, demographic variables of those covered (disability, veterans, low literacy, racial or ethnic minority, rural, over age 60), and households lacking broadband and personal computers. Find the tool at this link or via an internet search: https://www.census.gov/library/stories/2022/05/mapping-digital-equity-in-every-state.html.
10. *Cross-Reference Bandwidth Maps, State Requirements, HPSA, and Counseling Compact.* Have CITs examine all four constructs, looking for ways in which internet bandwidth, state licensing requirements, HPSA, and the Counseling Compact create opportunities and barriers for marginalized clients to access TMH.

Sample Lesson: Multicultural Counseling in the Digital World

Ming-hui Li, EdD, LMHC, LPC
St. John's University

Lesson Objectives

After this lesson, students will 1) learn the relationship between multicultural counseling and the digital world, 2) learn the importance of developing counselor multicultural competence in the digital world, and 3) learn principles for conducting digital multicultural counseling.

2024 CACREP Standards

Section 3.B (Social and cultural identities and experiences) and Standard 3.E.5 (The application of technology related to counseling).

Preparation Required

Students/trainees learned multicultural counseling competence models in a previous class.

Time Required for Lesson Delivery

The lesson is estimated to last one hour.

Structure and Audience for Lessons

This lesson can be conducted in-person or online synchronously. The audience of the lesson is doctoral students or counselors-in-training.

Lesson Content and Instructional Strategies

1. *Introduction:* The instructor begins by explaining the lesson's purpose, which is to effectively teach students how to conduct multicultural counseling sessions in a digital environment. Discuss the increasing reliance on technology in our daily lives and how this has affected how we communicate and seek support. Technology illiteracy may cause a marginalized minority group.
2. *Define multicultural counseling:* Discuss the concept of multicultural counseling, including the importance of understanding and respecting the cultural backgrounds, beliefs, and values of clients from diverse backgrounds. Emphasize the role of cultural

humility in building trust and rapport with clients from different cultural backgrounds.

3. *The benefits and challenges of digital counseling:* Discuss the benefits of digital counseling, including the convenience and accessibility it offers to clients and the potential for increased privacy and anonymity. The instructor, however, also highlights the challenges of digital counseling, including issues with technology and internet connectivity and the potential for misunderstandings and miscommunications due to the lack of social cues typically seen in person-to-person interactions.
4. *Digital modalities used in multicultural counseling:* Class discussion on and sharing experiences using TMH modalities such as video conferencing, smartphone apps, discussion forums, phone counseling, blogs, wikis, and podcasts.
5. *Multicultural competent counselor in the digital world:* The instructor discusses the importance for counselors to match our skills and competencies to embrace the new social context of our clients (in-person and through the internet). Counselors are not only individuals but also members of a global community. Certain technologies make it more possible to advocate with our clients or for clients to advocate for themselves. Technologies may provide specific benefits to members of marginalized or disenfranchised groups. In addition, using interactive media with marginalized or disenfranchised populations may allow them to connect to others in ways they may not have been able to face-to-face.
6. *Principles for conducting digital multicultural counseling:* The instructor provides students with principles for conducting multicultural counseling sessions in a digital environment, including tips for creating a comfortable and confidential space, maintaining boundaries, and addressing technical issues. Emphasize the importance of building rapport and establishing trust with clients, even when communicating remotely.
7. *Conclusion:* Summarize the key points covered in the lesson and encourage students to continue practicing and refining their skills in multicultural digital counseling. Remind them to stay current on the latest developments in technology and digital culture and be mindful of the unique challenges and opportunities of conducting multicultural counseling in a digital environment.

Assessment of Objectives

Correct answers are marked with an asterisk *

1. When conducting multicultural counseling, why is it important to consider the digitalization of the world?
   a. Digitalization is a fad
   b. Digitalization has turned the world into a unified culture—the digital culture
   c. Face-to-face relationships are no longer important
   d. Digitalization plays a role in our ways of life, regardless of cultural background *
2. Which of the following is NOT related to developing multicultural counseling competence in a digital world?
   a. Counselors improve skills and competencies to embrace the new social context of clients (in-person and through the internet)
   b. Counselors learn to use technology to connect and communicate with a marginalized population
   c. Counselors are not aware that technology has influenced their lives *
   d. Counselors know the benefits and limitations of using technology to conduct multicultural counseling
3. Which principles are inappropriate for conducting multicultural counseling in a digital world?
   a. Create a comfortable and confidential space
   b. Maintain appropriate boundaries
   c. * Employ the most advanced technology in the counseling process without assessing the client's capability of using such technology
   d. Addressing technical issues

Additional Resources

Goss, S., Anthony, K., Stretch, L. S., Nagel, D. M. (2016). *Technology in mental health: Application in practice, supervision, and training* (2nd ed.). Thomas.

Lee, C. C. (Ed.) (2019). *Multicultural issues in counseling: New approaches to diversity* (5th ed.). American Counseling Association.

Lui, J. H. L., Marcus, D. K., & Barry, C. T. (2017). Evidence-based apps? A review of mental health mobile applications in a psychotherapy context. *Professional Psychology: Research and Practice, 48*(3), 199–210. http://doi.org/10.1037/pro0000122

Robertson, H. (2021). *Telemental health and distance counseling: A counselor's guide to decisions, resources, and practice*. Springer.

Sample Lesson: Examining Cultural Counseling Directories and Services

Michael Jones, PhD, LPC-S, NCC, BC-TMH, University of the Cumberlands

Lesson Objectives

After this lesson, students will have

1) explored online directories and resources aimed at identifying cultural counseling services for clients,
2) critically examined these resources,
3) discussed the risks and benefits of recommending or referring diverse clients to these resources, and
4) create a directory list with the pros and cons of the websites (accessibility, ease of use).

2024 CACREP Standards

Section 3.B (Social and Cultural Identities and Experiences) and 3.E.5 (The application of technology related to counseling).

Materials and/or Technology Required

Internet access and a mechanism to capture information discovered during activity. For in-person classes, at least one student in the group or pair must access the internet via a device. Online synchronous classes require an internet and video platform to deliver instruction. Asynchronous classes require internet and a learning management system (LMS) with discussion board capabilities.

Preparation Required

Students should have prior instruction on multicultural counseling and the impact of TMH on social and cultural diversity. Instructors may wish to review some of the sites listed in the resources in preparation for the lesson. Instructors should emphasize the importance of addressing multicultural populations with resources that provide care from a diversity, equity, justice, and inclusion standpoint that also informs anti-racist practice.

Estimated Time Required for Lesson Delivery

Prior instructional time may vary; the lesson can be delivered in approximately 45–60 minutes.

Structure and Audience for Lesson

Graduate students in counselor education. The lesson can be delivered in-person, online synchronously, or online asynchronously.

Lesson Content and Instructional Strategies

1. *Understanding Cultural Counseling Directories and Services.* The instructor begins by describing the purpose of cultural counseling directories and services, explaining that these services allow individuals from specific cultural communities to find counselors who specialize in specific cultural groups or share similar cultural characteristics, such as race, language, sexuality, or religion. In some cases, directories are published by professional organizations where the public can locate counselors who share or support their identity. In other cases, specific counseling services are marketed to a particular population (e.g., Betterhelp's Pride Counseling or Faith Counseling).
2. *Exploring online services and directories.* Students are asked to work individually, in pairs, or in small groups to research online cultural counseling directories and services. Students can search any terms or combination, for example, "counseling for Asian communities," "LGBTQ-affirming counseling," or other terms. Students are encouraged to search for various cultural characteristics—age, race, gender, religion, disability status, sexuality—and try to identify specialized services or directories for counseling for that population.

3. *Critical examination of resources.* For each source located, students critically examine the website by asking the following questions:
   a. What is the source of this service/directory? Is it managed by a professional organization or a reputable source?
   b. How easy was it to locate the site?
   c. What are the qualifications of the counselors? What specific training or experiences do they have in relation to the cultural community?
   d. How does a counselor join the directory or service? Is there information on the site for licensed counselors who wish to join?
   e. Is there any information on telemental health on the site? If so, what?
   f. How would a viewer be able to authenticate if the source is a professional counseling site? Are there any links to the site's licensing organizations or the counselor's credentialing organizations?
   g. Where are these therapists located? Are there any in your state or a state with the Counseling Compact?
   h. Is the site easily accessible to individuals with disabilities?
   i. What else do you notice about the source, if anything?
4. *Discussion of risks and benefits.* The instructor then leads the group in a discussion to share what they found. Students share information from at least one site based on a cultural identity group. If possible, student groups share from as many different identity groups as possible. The instructor then leads a discussion on the risks and benefits of referring clients to the sites they found. Students are asked to share their thoughts on the following questions:
   a. How might the resources on this site be helpful or harmful to a client?
   b. What more would I need to know about this site before recommending it to a client or using it as a referral source?

Assessment of Objectives

The information students gathered for each site can be evaluated to determine whether it aligns with the criteria outlined in items A–D above. Similarly, online asynchronous students can share their results on a discussion board where peers comment on the risks and benefits of the information found. The grading of the discussion board can serve as an assessment measure.

Additional Resources

Sample directories/services:

- Asian American Federation Mental Health Directory: https://mhd.aafederation.org/
- AFSP Mental Health for Marginalized Communities: https://afsp.org/mental-health-resources-for-marginalized-communities/
- Clinicians of Color: https://www.cliniciansofcolor.org/
- Gay Therapy Center: https://www.thegaytherapycenter.com/
- Pink Therapy: https://pinktherapy.com/
- Psychotherapy Today: https://www.psychologytoday.com/
- The JED Foundation Therapy Resources: https://jedfoundation.org/therapy-resources/
- Therapy for Black Girls: https://therapyforblackgirls.com/
- Therapy for Black Men: https://therapyforblackmen.org/

5

Lifespan Development

Lifespan development encompasses growth and changes in human beings, from birth through death, in traits such as physical, cognitive, emotional, moral, sexual, personality, cultural, and others. The 2016 version of the Council for Accreditation of Counseling and Related Educational Programs (CACREP; 2015) standards refers to this content area as "Human Growth and Development," while the 2024 standards refer to it as "Lifespan Development" (CACREP, 2024) Other terms include "psychosocial development" or "development across the lifespan." Most instructors would agree that counselors-in-training (CITs) must understand the growth and development of students and clients across the lifespan, but not all would agree that telemental health (TMH) should be included in lifespan development training. In a survey of 74 counselor educators, educators were asked which CACREP areas they taught included content on TMH. None of the 74 educators surveyed (n = 0) indicated that they included content on TMH in a course on human growth and development (Robertson & Lowell, 2021).

Telemental health is being utilized with clients across the lifespan. Counselors need different skills to deliver TMH services to clients at different learning stages with different developmental ages and cognitive abilities. In addition, technology impacts individual growth and development in these areas. Thus, it is recommended that instructors focus not only on the use of TMH counseling at various developmental stages but also on the overall impact of technology on an individual's growth and development. Instructors need to train CITs not only on how to utilize TMH at various developmental stages but also on how technology impacts development. This chapter aims to assist the instructor in identifying key components of lifespan development that CITs need in their training and practice of TMH.

Key Concepts

CACREP Standards

The connection between lifespan development and TMH practice is not as direct as in other areas of counselor training. However, the review of the CACREP standards below demonstrates how TMH can be infused into lifespan development training. Table 5.1 provides suggestions on integrating TMH content with these standards. If these concepts are unfamiliar, the instructor is encouraged to explore the training and reading materials suggested in Chapter 1.

Table 5.1

CACREP Section 3.C (Lifespan Development) and Suggested TMH Content

CACREP Standards (2024)	Suggested TMH Content
CACREP Standards (2024)	Suggested TMH Content
3.C.1. Theories of individual and family development across the lifespan.	Understanding generational differences regarding technology and its use (see below).
3.C.2. Theories of cultural identity development.	Application of TMH to diverse populations (see Chapter 4).
3.C.3. Theories of learning.	Appropriate use of TMH based on an individual's cognitive ability, including their use and familiarity with technology; pros/cons of technology on learning (Courage et al., 2015; Globokar, 2018; Molnar et al., 2021).
3.C.4. Theories of personality and psychological development.	Impact of technology on an individual's ability to develop patience, empathy, and kindness (Globokar, 2018)

CACREP Standards (2024)	Suggested TMH Content
3.C.5. Theories and neurobiological etiology of addictions.	Exploring technology as addiction; lack of a DSM diagnosis in internet addiction; use of TMH in treating technology-related process addictions (see Chapter 11).
3.C.6. Structures for affective relationships, bonds, couples, marriages, and families.	Application of TMH to couples and families (see Chapter 16).
3.C.7. Models of resilience, optimal development, and wellness in individuals and families across the lifespan.	Impact of technology, including social media, on social/emotional wellness (see below).
3.C.8. Models of psychosocial adjustment and adaptation to illness and disability.	Application of TMH to people with disabilities (see Chapter 14).
3.C.9. The role of sexual development and sexuality related to overall wellness.	Examining the AASECT Code of Conduct (2020) and TMH; pros and cons of sex education via the internet/technology (Tylka & Cook-Cottone, 2016); **digisexuality** (McArthur & Twist, 2017); role of technology in sexual development.
3.C.10. Biological, neurological, and physiological factors that affect lifespan development, functioning, behavior, resilience, and overall wellness.	American Academy of Pediatrics (AAP) recommendations for technology use in children (AAP, 2016).
3.C.11. Systemic, cultural, and environmental factors that affect lifespan development, functioning, behavior, resilience, and overall wellness.	Propensity for TMH to increase access to treatment for diverse populations, yet systemic barriers/digital divide (see Chapter 4).
3.C.12. the influence of mental and physical health conditions on coping, resilience, and overall wellness for individuals and families across the lifespan.	Impact of technology, including social media, on social/emotional wellness (see below).
3.C.13. Effects of crises, disasters, stress, grief, and trauma across the lifespan.	Impact of technology and TMH services (e.g., hotlines, text lines, warmlines) in providing crisis support (Goss & Ferns, 2016).

Generational Differences and TMH Use

An instructor is responsible for correcting inaccuracies or falsely held beliefs about the practice of TMH. When TMH first emerged, one common myth was the concern that TMH could not be used with certain age groups. People doubted its ability to be effective with children and worried that older adults might be unable to utilize the required technology. TMH has been effective with older adults and has been specifically used to reduce elder abuse (Bitondo Dyer et al., 2020). However, research indicates that internet and computer use decline with age (Pew Research Group, 2019; Siren & Knudsen, 2016). Learning new computer skills is often linked to employment benefits, which may be less motivating for older adults no longer in the workforce (Hargittai & Dobransky, 2017). Internet access and computer use are lower among those with lower socioeconomic status (Pew Research, 2021), which may include older adults who are already out of the workforce and on a fixed income.

Children and adolescents have had effective outcomes utilizing TMH with various counseling services (Comer et al., 2017; McCarty et al., 2015; Stephan et al., 2016). During the COVID-19 pandemic, children and adolescents received all educational instruction via technology, primarily video conferencing software. While many students have become accustomed to this technology, there is growing concern that long-term digital learning, outside of a live classroom environment, has impacted children's social-emotional growth and academic development (Molnar et al., 2021). TMH can provide benefits and challenges to clients with focus and attention issues. Small children, for example, may struggle with focus and attention, as well as people with cognitive disabilities or certain medical conditions. Video and visual imagery may help engage the client in the session and maintain attention by providing visual cues or images, videos, sharing screens, or even using whiteboard features on specific software platforms.

Social Media and Social-Emotional Wellness

Social media includes a variety of platforms, such as Instagram, Threads, Facebook, Snapchat, LinkedIn, and others. Social media brings people together, and users can post almost anything they wish while also creating a digital footprint. People, particularly young people, have a limited understanding of how their digital footprint can create negative impressions for friends, family, partners, employers, and colleagues. Clients may be concerned that online counseling will leave a digital footprint and/or that the content of sessions may be accessible online.

Counseling ethical codes strictly prohibit counselors from posting confidential information to social media platforms (ACA, 2014; NBCC, 2023).

Another concern with social media is that a **poster's** online persona may not accurately portray their true identity. While there is not necessarily direct harm in someone inflating, fabricating, or falsifying their online profile, there are concerns surrounding the safety of minors and the potential for the predatory behavior of online adults. Even when there is no malicious intent on the part of the poster, individuals often compare their own experiences to others online. A poster's friendships, social events, videos, and images may be altered to appear more desirable to the public and to attract more attention (e.g., "likes" and "shares"). People (both children and adults) often compare their lives to others on social media, which can have negative consequences on emotional well-being and contribute to conditions such as eating disorders (Donovan, 2024) or depression (Cruz et al., 2022).

There are concerns that social media and technology will adversely impact social development. Technology has been praised for helping affinity groups connect with others at great distances who share their passions and interests. Yet, there are concerns that technology contributes to exclusionary and isolating behavior, impacting social and emotional well-being. Numerous examples exist of people being cruel, deceitful, vengeful, and predatory to others via technology, including instances of discrimination (Zeligmari et al., 2022), as the device (e.g., computer, tablet, phone) provides a false sense of anonymity to the perpetrator of these behaviors. Many clients are accustomed to being behind a screen for work, school, or social reasons. Clients may have previously experienced unsafe online settings where the individual they interacted with was not supportive or trustworthy. CITs need to overcome those preconceived notions and build trusted, genuine, and empathic relationships with clients via TMH.

Teaching Techniques

Connecting TMH to lifespan development may appear more challenging than other topics in counselor education. As a reminder, instructors can explore the use of TMH across developmental stages and the impact of technology on development. Below are some suggested strategies for integrating these principles into the curriculum. These strategies utilize the andragogical principles discussed in Chapter 2, including self-motivated learning, using prior experiences, recognizing a need for information, and immediately applying knowledge in a real-world context (Knowles, 1975).

1. *Reexamining Foundational Theories.* Lifespan theories, such as those of Piaget and Erikson, were created long before technology use in counseling practice. Some researchers suggest we seek opportunities to connect technology to these theoretical foundations (Pea & Cole, 2019). Have CITs examine these theories using a technological lens and share their results. Some questions for CITs to consider: How might these theories be different if technology was present during their development? How might I need to consider my theoretical approach differently with clients and students when using TMH?
2. *Social Media Age Limits.* Have CITs explore the "fine print" of social media use policies, looking for information such as age limits, parental permissions, or other restrictions. Have students explore how or why these policies are relevant, if at all, and how these platforms might impact individual development.
3. *Screentime and Children.* Examine the American Academy of Pediatrics's (AAP) recommendations for screen time and other behaviors such as sleep and exercise/play time (https://www.healthychildren.org/). Have CITs explore their thoughts/beliefs on the feasibility of these guidelines. How might parental status (e.g., employment, socioeconomic, marital) impact one's ability to maintain such guidelines?
4. *Using TMH Across the Lifespan.* Ask CITs to create fictional case studies of clients needing counseling at various developmental stages, including childhood, adolescence, young adulthood, middle adulthood, and later adulthood. Include the presenting problem(s), present functioning, and living environment. Have CITs explore the use of TMH with each case and determine what special considerations would need to be addressed before engaging in TMH treatment.
5. *Using TMH With Minors.* Counseling with minors, whether F2F or TMH, requires specific considerations. CITs can explore TMH considerations for working with minors, informed by the ACA and NBCC Codes of Ethics.
6. *Benefits and Positive Contributions of Social Media and the Internet.* Many cases are available in the news where the internet, social media, and online connections have supported someone's personal, social, and emotional development. Have CITs explore and

discuss these examples (or their own) and how TMH, counselors, or social policies could foster continued efforts toward growth development.

7. *Danger and Damage of Social Media and the Internet.* Many cases are available in the news on the damage inflicted upon people's personal, social, and emotional development via the internet. Have CITs explore and discuss these examples (or their own) and how TMH, counselors, or social policies could help.
8. *Sexuality and Technology.* Explore concepts such as **AImorosexuality** (Albalat Peraita, 2023)**, digisexuality (**McArthur & Twist, 2017), and **teledildonics (**Knowles, 2017). Have CITs consider the following: "To what extent am I familiar with these concepts and their role in sexual development? How do they vary from other, more common sexual technologies, such as dating apps or online pornography? How can I be an affirming provider for individuals who use technology in their sexual development?"
9. *Technology and Brain Development.* Explore recent research on the use of technology and brain development. Have CITs share what they've found in their research, the source(s) of their research, and its potential impact on individual development or the use of TMH.
10. *Personal Technology Audit and Overall Wellness.* Have CITs estimate how many hours per day they spend on technology or their devices, such as phones, tablets, and laptops. Have them record their daily estimations (e.g., hours, minutes) on email, texting, social media, gaming, video, or other platforms. CITs can discuss the pros and cons of their own technology use and how it impacts their overall wellness. Some devices allow users to check their use through features on the device, which CITs can use to see how accurate their estimations were regarding their use of technology.

Sample Lesson: Observing the Impact of Technology Across the Lifespan

James Bethea, PhD, LMHC, CRC
St. John's University

Lesson Objectives

At the end of this lesson, students will

1) evaluate technological use in multiple age groups,
2) discuss the potential impact of that technology on individual development, including learning, cultural, personality, psychological, and sexual development, and
3) make theoretical connections to observations in a practical sense.

2024 CACREP Standards

Section 3.C (Lifespan Development), Standards 3.C.1 (Individual and family development), 3.C.2 (Cultural identity development), 3.C.3 (Learning), 3.C.4 (Personality and psychological development), 3.C.9 (Role of sexual development and sexuality related to overall wellness).

Preparation Required

Students are provided with prior instruction in lifespan development topics/theories, as well as the impact of technology on lifespan development. Students are provided with the assignment below prior to classroom discussion and activity.

Estimated Time Required for Lesson Delivery

Prior instruction time may vary. Time for this activity is approximately 45–60 minutes.

Structure and Audience for Lesson

This activity is designed for in-person or online instruction, including master's, doctoral, or professional development training. Online asynchronous instruction can utilize discussion boards to facilitate group dialogue that would normally occur during live instruction.

Lesson Content and Instructional Strategies

1. The instructor provides prior content on lifespan development, including cognitive, physical, moral, social-emotional, cultural, and sexual development.
2. The instructor provides prior content on the impact of technology on individual development. The instructor can utilize the content and resources discussed in this book to support instruction.
3. Students are provided with the assignment below within their syllabus or as a supplemental learning activity:

   Observing the Impact of Technology Across the Lifespan

   a. You will visit three public places (e.g., library, shopping center, coffee shop, park) at three separate times, spending a minimum of one hour at each location.
   b. You will observe individuals from separate age groups at each location, loosely categorized as children, adolescents, young adults, middle adults, and older adults. For each setting, focus on at least two age groups to report on (a total of six observations).
   c. During your observation, you are specifically observing their use of technology in that setting. Technology may include phones, laptops, tablets, smartphones, smartwatches, gaming devices, or any other items you would classify as technology.
   d. Record your response to the following questions: 1) What is happening in the public place? Describe the setting, surroundings, and events. 2) What is the person/people doing at this location? What do you think brought them here (e.g., work, leisure, task)? 3) How are they using technology? Describe the technology they are using and how they are using it. 4) How are they interacting with others, if at all? To what extent does their technology impact their interaction? 5) What theoretical connections (from prior readings) can you make to your observation(s)? 6) What other general observations do you make?
   e. Students will record their responses to these questions for each group they observe at each site. Note: the instructor determines the format for the student response (e.g., paper, journal, discussion board) and specifies these instructions in advance for students.

4. When students have completed the assignment, the instructor facilitates a group dialogue with students. This dialogue can occur in a large group (classroom), small groups (3–5 students in a group), or in pairs. If teaching online synchronously, the instructor can create breakout rooms for small groups or paired discussions and utilize the chat feature for large group discussions. During the discussion, the instructor poses the following questions:
   a. Based on the developmental models we have discussed in class, what stages of development did you notice among the groups you observed? You should specifically address the theoretical development models in multiple areas (e.g., cognitive, social).
   b. What connections do you make to the person/group's development and use of technology? For example, how might their use of technology be different if they were at a different stage of development (again, consider development from multiple perspectives, e.g., learning, cultural, personality, psychological, and sexual development)? Were there any theoretical constructs "brought to life" as a result of your observation(s)?
   c. How essential is/was technology to the situations you observed? If the technology did not exist, how would the person or situation be different?
   d. How might our observation, assessment, and awareness of technology and individual development impact our relationship with clients and students during counseling? How can we support clients and students in using technology for healthy development?

Assessment of Objectives

Assessment of the lesson objective will be via the classroom discussion/dialogue and the student's response to the activity. Students may also be asked to reference this activity in a reflective journal or other assignment.

Sample Lesson: Detoxing from Our Digital Lifeline

Brittany L. Prioleau, PhD, LCMHC, NCC
Mercer University

Lesson Objectives

At the end of this lesson, students will

1) define and recognize signs of digital dependence,
2) understand the impact of digital dependence on mental and physical health,
3) identify strategies for a digital detox and its potential benefits, and) develop a personal digital detox plan.

2024 CACREP Standards

Section 3.C (Lifespan Development), Standards 3.C.5 (Theories and neurobiological etiology of addictions), 3.C.7 (Models of resilience, optimal development, and wellness in individuals and families across the lifespan).

Materials and/or Technology Required

1) Students need a laptop, tablet, or smartphone; students may use several devices for this activity.
2) Handout of DSM-5-TR general criteria for substance use disorder.
3) SAMHSA wellness model (see resources).

Preparation Required

Students are provided with prior instruction in lifespan development topics, as well as the impact of technology on lifespan development. The instructor should introduce the digital detox activity the week before the lesson (see instructions below).

Estimated Time Required for Lesson Delivery

The experiential activity will occur for the duration of the class time (e.g., 2–3 hours).

Structure and Audience for Lesson

This activity is designed for in-person instruction. The intended audience is master's students enrolled in counseling programs. The lesson can be adapted to online synchronous instruction.

Lesson Content and Instructional Strategies

1. Introduction (15 minutes)
   a. *Icebreaker Activity (5 minutes):* Begin with a brief icebreaker to engage students and introduce the topic of electronic dependence. Have students remove all digital or electronic devices for the remainder of the class. Ask students to share their favorite digital activities and discuss their reasons for using them.
   b. *Class Discussion (10 minutes):* Facilitate a discussion on the concept of digital dependence. Ask questions like: What is digital dependence? How do you know if you are digitally dependent? How is digital dependence like other forms of dependence? Can digital dependence have negative effects on our lives?
2. *Understanding Digital Dependence Presentation (15 minutes):* Provide information on the signs and symptoms of digital dependence. Use examples and statistics to highlight the prevalence and impact of excessive digital use on mental and physical health. Provide examples of how technology can be used beneficially.
3. *Strategies for Digital Detox (25 minutes):*
   a. *Presentation (10 minutes):* Introduce various strategies for a digital detox, including setting boundaries establishing electronic-free zones.
   b. *Interactive Activity (15 minutes):* Have students brainstorm and share ideas for a digital detox plan. Encourage creativity and emphasize personalized approaches.
4. *Creating Personal Digital Detox Plans (25 minutes):*
   a. *Individual Reflection (10 minutes):* Ask students to reflect on their digital usage habits and identify areas where they may need a digital detox.
   b. *Guided Activity (15 minutes):* Provide a template for students to create their own digital detox plans. Emphasize setting realistic goals and the importance of gradual changes.

5. *Discussion/Reflection (15 minutes):* Toward the end of class, the instructor engages the class in group discussion to reflect on not using technology during class. Some prompting questions may include:
   a. What physical sensations did you notice, if any, being unable to use your technology? How were they impacted, if at all, by being able to see your phone?
   b. What emotional and cognitive responses did you have while separated from technology? How might you feel different if you weren't informed last week and the detox was unplanned?
   c. How long do you think you could go without using any technology? This exercise was only an hour long. How would you do with an evening, day, week, month, or longer?
   d. Look at the DSM-5 general criteria for substance use disorder (SUD). Currently, there is no DSM-5-TR diagnosis for technology, internet, or gaming addiction. What are your thoughts on that? Do you think there should be? Why or why not?
   e. How might technology impact student/client wellness and development? How can counselors help them use technology for healthy development in all areas of wellness?
   f. What other observations or takeaways have you gleaned from this activity?
6. *Conclusion and Homework Assignment (10 minutes):*
   a. *Summary (5 minutes):* Summarize key points from the lesson.
   b. *Homework Assignment (5 minutes):* Assign students to implement their digital detox plans for a longer period of time (e.g., a weekend) and journal their experiences. They will share their reflections in the next class.

Instructions

1. The instructor introduces the assignment to students at the close of the week prior so students are prepared in advance. The digital experiment will last for the duration of the class period.
2. *Digital Detox Assignment:* Read aloud: "We will be engaging in a digital detoxification activity next week. During next week's class, students will not use technology. Students may not use their smartphones, laptops, tablets, smartwatches, or other electronic devices. Students will be required to place their phones on a table

in the front of the classroom and to place backpacks with tablets, laptops, smartwatches, and devices under their chairs or in the back of the room. Please notify members of your family, work, and other key people that you will not be accessible during class. Come prepared with other materials, such as a notebook, pen, pencil, or paper."

3. During the digital detox class period, the instructor reminds students to put their phones in the front of the room and all laptops and devices beneath the chairs or in the back of the room.
4. The instructor teaches a class/lesson for at least 60–90 minutes, using NO TECHNOLOGY. The instructor utilizes lectures, small group work, role-playing, dry-erase board, chart paper/markers, or other non-technological learning materials. Learning games, icebreakers, and manipulatives also foster learning, but some instructional content should be delivered. Students should not be allowed to access their technology during class.

Assessment of Objectives

Assessment of the lesson objective will be assessed via classroom discussion/dialogue and the students' response to the activity. *Option:* Create a homework assignment where students try a detox for more extended periods and discuss the activity in a reflective journal of the assignment.

References

American Psychiatric Association. (2022). *Diagnostic and statistical manual of mental disorders* (5th ed., text rev.).

Substance Abuse and Mental Health Services Administration (SAMHSA). (2016). *Learn the eight dimensions of wellness.* https://store.samhsa.gov/sites/default/files/sma16-4953.pdf

Sample Handout

Adapted from DSM-5 (APA, 2013).

General criteria for addictive disorders include:

A problematic pattern of ___________ use leading to clinically significant impairment or distress, as manifested by at least two of the following occurring within a 12-month period:

1. ___________ often taken in larger amounts or over a longer period of time than intended.
2. A persistent desire or unsuccessful efforts to cut down or control ___________ use.
3. A great deal of time is spent in activities necessary to obtain ___________, use ___________, or recover from its effects.
4. Craving or a strong desire to use ___________.
5. Recurrent ___________ use resulting in failure to fulfill major obligations at work, school, or home.
6. Continued ___________ use despite having persistent or recurrent social or interpersonal problems caused or exacerbated by the use of ___________.
7. Important social, occupational, or recreational activities are given up or reduced because of ___________ use.
8. Recurrent ___________ use in situations in which it is physically hazardous.
9. ___________ use is continued despite knowledge of having persistent or recurring physical or psychological problems likely exacerbated by ___________ use.
10. Tolerance
11. Withdrawal

Note: Insert any technology in the space before "use," including internet, gaming, social media, texting, scrolling, watching videos, or other activities.

6

Career Development

Career development is a multifaceted concept. Brown (2016) shares a preference for Sears's (1982) definition of career development, "a lifelong process involving psychological, sociological, educational, economic, and physical factors as well as chance factors that interact to influence the career of an individual" (Brown, 2016, p. 8). Brown argues that culture plays a significant role in career development, as does the emergence of technology. Brown posits that career theorists discussed the use of technology and its impact on career development services well before COVID-19 and the telemental health (TMH) movement.

The origins of career development within the profession are well-known by instructors and counselors-in-training (CITs), dating back to Frank Parsons and his Breadwinner's Institute of Boston in 1905 (Brown, 2016). Instructors and CITs may not realize that career development was one of the first counseling specializations to embrace technology into practice. While I use the term TMH in this chapter, career development is an area of counseling that may not include mental health in its scope of practice. The term's usage may not accurately describe the work of career professionals. While career concerns can result in emotional or mental health issues, the practitioner focuses on career concerns.

Key Concepts

CACREP Standards

Career development is both a core curricular area and a specialization within the CACREP curriculum. It is also one of the few areas of the CACREP standards that has historically included the use of technology. Table 6.1 provides examples of how TMH can be infused into career development training. If concepts are unfamiliar, the instructor is encouraged to explore the training and reading materials suggested in Chapter 1.

Table 6.1

CACREP Section 3.D (Career Development) and Suggested TMH Content

CACREP Standards (2024)	Suggested TMH Content
3.D.1. Theories and models of career development, counseling, and decision-making.	Exploration of how career theories and models can be adapted for and impacted by TMH delivery.
3.D.2. Approaches for conceptualizing the interrelationships among and between work, socioeconomic standing, wellness, disability, trauma, relationships, and other life roles and factors.	Clarify understanding of career practitioner's role, e.g., career counseling and/or career services, and the importance of this clarification for ethical TMH client treatment.
3.D.3. Processes for identifying and using career, avocational, educational, occupational, and labor market information resources, technology, and information systems.	Understanding geographic job markets when using TMH for career counseling; capacity to access labor market information online (e.g., Department of Labor, Bureau of Labor Statistics).
3.D.4. Approaches for assessing the conditions of the work environment on clients' life experiences.	Experience with online career information systems (e.g., O*Net, etc.) and using such systems when delivering TMH services.
3.D.5. Strategies for assessing abilities, interests, values, personality, and other factors that contribute to career development.	Use of computer-assisted career assessments (Osborn et al., 2019); emergence of computer-assisted guidance systems (CAGS) (Harris-Bowlsbey & Sampson, 2005).

CACREP Standards (2024)	Suggested TMH Content
3.D.6. Career development program planning, organization, implementation, administration, and evaluation.	Strategies and cautions for implementing online career programming and services (Sampson & Lenz, 2023).
3.D.7. Developmentally responsive strategies for empowering individuals to engage in culturally sustaining career and educational development and employment opportunities.	Developmentally and culturally appropriate responses to delivering career services virtually (see Chapters 4 and 5).
3.D.8. Strategies for advocating for employment support for individuals facing barriers in the workplace.	Capacity for TMH to create access to career services; the need to overcome barriers based on inequities to access TMH career services (see Chapters 4 and 14).
3.D.9. Strategies for facilitating client skill development for career, educational, and life-work planning and management.	Modeling TMH career sessions with clients and students; observing CITs provide TMH instruction on career management tools.
3.D.10. Career and postsecondary training readiness and educational decision-making.	Using online information to support clients and students in postsecondary career planning; capacity for TMH to facilitate and/or observe client/student learning.
3.D.11. Strategies for improving access to educational and occupational opportunities for people from marginalized groups.	Awareness of systemic barriers, including the digital divide, to access career and educational opportunities; advocacy efforts for technology access for marginalized populations.
3.D.12. Ethical and legal issues relevant to career development and career counseling.	Examining the NCDA Code of Ethics, specifically Section F (NCDA, 2024), and NCDA position statement on social networking (NCDA, 2015).

Career Counseling Versus Career Planning Services

Providing career development services does not typically require a state license or certification. Unlike other counseling specializations such as mental health, school counseling, or addictions counseling, career development does not usually require state-level licensure or certification. The lack of state-level licensure means that career professionals providing services via TMH may practice across state lines unless statutes prohibit such practice. This is positive for the provider because they can serve more clients with fewer limitations. However, state-level counseling licensure allows professional counselors to bill insurance or will enable clients to seek recourse if they are harmed. Without a counseling license or certification, clients must pay directly for services, which creates barriers for clients without financial means. Additionally, if career practitioners become aware of a mental health concern, they cannot ethically treat that concern without a counseling license. Those cases need to be referred to a qualified provider, which creates a disruption in services for the client.

The issue of mental health requires clarification of the terms *career counseling* and *career planning services*. NCDA defines these terms as follows:

> "Career planning" services include an active provision of information designed to help a client with a specific need, such as review of a resume; assistance in networking strategies; identification of occupations based on values, interests, skills, prior work experience, and/or other characteristics; support in the job-seeking process; and assessment by means of paper-based and/or online inventories of interest, abilities, personality, work-related values, and/or other characteristics. ... "Career counseling" provides the opportunity for a deeper level of involvement with the client, based on establishing a professional counseling relationship and the potential for assisting clients with career and personal development concerns beyond those included in career planning. (NCDA, 2024, p. 3)

These two definitions exemplify the potential for career planning and counseling to become blurred. Career practitioners must use caution not to engage in counseling unless qualified to offer such services. The professional must make ethical decisions to refer as needed.

The lack of state license or certification creates risks of ethical violations. A state licensing and certification board is responsible for reviewing violations, conducting hearings, and making decisions on disciplinary actions. While similar administrative and disciplinary processes exist for national certifications, those credentials are optional, and the outcome of disciplinary measures may hold less weight than at the state level. Career professionals should provide information on national certifications to clients, as well as information on filing grievances. While a lack of state-level licensure or certification can increase access, particularly when using TMH mediums, it also risks a lack of oversight and financial burdens.

Online Career Information

The U.S. Bureau of Labor Statistics (BLS) has collected employment and industry data since the late 1800s and early 1900s. The BLS published the *Occupational Outlook Handbook* (OOH) in 1949 (U.S. BLS, 2019). The *Dictionary of Occupational Titles* (DOT) was published in 1939 (Brown, 2016). Fortunately, career information was transitioned online in the late 1990s and early 2000s when the O*NET replaced the DOT. O*NET is a digital database that can expand to accommodate the growing and changing workforce, a welcome contrast to the static printed materials in the DOT (Mariani, 1999).

Online information includes data from the O*NET and OOH, job postings, employer information, online networking, career and employer research, and other tools. Many elements of career development utilize online tools, making TMH ideal for career development services. Even basic strategies like job application completion are often done online. TMH career professionals can work directly with clients to explore career information through online tools. Yet, finding career information online can also come with risks. Career professionals have a responsibility to help clients identify information that is reputable and valid. Engaging in the virtual career development process with a professional in real-time makes clients less likely to be victims of fraudulent activities. A career professional can coach clients to recognize cues of potential schemes during live virtual sessions. Career professionals practicing online can demonstrate how to research employers through the employer's website, public records, and documents, verifying the security of websites where candidates are asked to enter information. Instructors and CITs can brainstorm potential red flags or triggers that indicate suspected fraudulent or unethical activity in online information.

Teaching Techniques

Instructors can introduce the issues of career development via TMH in a variety of ways. Below is a list of suggested strategies that might reinforce or supplement CITs' understanding of TMH and career development. These strategies utilize the andragogical principles addressed in previous chapters, including self-motivated learning, using prior experiences, recognizing a need for information, and immediately applying learning in a real-world context (Knowles, 1975).

1. *Comparing NCDA, NECA, and ACA Codes of Ethics.* Two primary career development organizations are the National Career Development Association (NCDA) and the National Employment Counseling Association (NECA). NECA specifies that its members adhere to the ACA Code of Ethics. Have CITs examine the *ACA Code of Ethics* (2014; specifically, Section H) and the *NCDA Code of Ethics* (2024; specifically, Section F). What variations and similarities exist between the two codes?
2. *Virtual Relationships.* The ACA Code of Ethics Standard A.5.e prohibits virtual relationships, whereas the NCDA Code of Ethics Section F.7.g requires fair and equitable social media policies. CITs can review these two standards and discuss how social media policies vary in career development and personal counseling contexts.
3. *Online Career Information.* Various career information tools exist online (e.g., O*Net, OOH). CITs can engage in mock TMH sessions with peers where they verbally explain, instruct, and model the use of these tools in an online session, using features such as **screen sharing**. Following the mock session, CITs share their strengths and challenges in conducting the career information session online.
4. *Geographic Differences in the Job Market.* The instructor can create fictional case studies of clients who desire to pursue specific careers in various regions of the country (e.g., a plumber in Chicago, an accountant in New Orleans, a nurse in Topeka). Have CITs use career information online from the BLS to research job market trends in that region for a particular career. Have CITs share their findings and struggles.
5. *Employment Rates and Internet Access.* In Chapter 4, CITs were encouraged to use the U.S. Census's "Digital Equity Act Population Viewer" to explore digital access in various regions. Have CITs cross reference BLS data and unemployment rates with digital access. Discuss how digital access can support/hinder accessing career counseling in that region.
6. *Online Career Assessments.* Various paid and free career assessments are available online. Have CITs engage in mock TMH sessions with peers, where CITs administer and review assessment results online using features such as screen sharing. Following the mock session, CITs can share their strengths and challenges

in conducting the online career assessment (see Chapter 9 for supporting information).

7. *Considering Culture in Career Development.* Most CITs learn elements of multicultural counseling in their program, including multicultural career counseling (Evans & Sejuit, 2021). Ask CITs to consider culture in the TMH delivery of career services. What cultural factors need to be considered, and how might we adapt services to accommodate culture when delivering career services via TMH?
8. *College Information.* Many school counselors help students explore college information. Have CITs share tools they could use, including paid and unpaid, to access college information. How might accessing these tools create or limit access to college information or other issues of equity?
9. *Red Flags for Online Career Information.* One of the risks of online information is its validity. Have CITs create a list of potential "red flags" or indicators that the career information may be inaccurate, invalid, or unsafe and share their results.
10. *Career Website Audit.* Have CITs select one website that contains information and conduct an audit of the site to determine its accuracy, validity, and safety. CITs can share what information they were able to find on the website's contributors and development, as well as the competence of those individuals to create career development information.

Sample Lesson: Transformational Learning in TMH – Finding a Life Through Career Development

Pamelia Brott, PhD, LPC, NCC, ACS

Career development is more than finding a job—it is about finding a life. The constructivist lens in narrative approaches provides opportunities for career counseling to focus on illuminating the client's story (Brott, 2017). Assessments hold value as cognitive tools to organize self-report information into models and frameworks that illuminate the story. Instead of matching the person to the job, clients can learn to co-construct life through experiences and meanings, to deconstruct life as contextual and informative, to reconstruct a mattering in life that is adaptable and sustainable, and to construct a prototype of the next chapters in finding a life. Various tools can be used to guide clients through the storied approach process (Brott, 2001).

Graduate students in CACREP counselor education programs are required to complete a career development curriculum containing theories, approaches, processes, strategies, and methods that are ethical and culturally relevant. Most of the curriculum delivery has focused on how to provide counseling in a face-to-face (F2F) format. However, the impact of COVID-19 on education, training, and counseling services has led to an abrupt shift from in-person to online delivery. This has challenged counselor educators to be innovative in training methods for knowledge and skill acquisition by graduate CITs that can accommodate virtual environments. Therefore, this lesson plan is about how to provide the knowledge and skills for articulating clients' personal narratives of finding a life through life roles by using the storied approach process in a virtual environment.

Lesson Objectives

At the end of this lesson, students will be able to:

1) Articulate constructivist theories in career development that relate a narrative-storied approach to career counseling,
2) Define career development in a culturally relevant perspective as "finding a life,"
3) Illustrate "finding a life" through life roles, and
4) Compose a personal narrative of "finding a life."

2024 CACREP Standards

Section 3.D (Career Development), Standards 3.D.1 (Theories and models of career development, counseling, and decision making), 3.D.2 (Approaches for conceptualizing the interrelationships among and between work, socioeconomic standing, wellness, disability, trauma, relationships, and other life roles and factors), 3.D.3 (Processes for identifying and using career, avocational, educational, occupational and labor market information resources, technology, and information systems), 3.D.5 (Strategies for assessing abilities, interests, values, personality, and other factors that contribute to career development), and 3.D.12 (Ethical and legal issues relevant to career development and career counseling).

Materials and/or Technology Required

Supplemental readings if the course textbook does not include constructivist approaches to career development, a computer, and access to video-based interaction (e.g., Zoom, Skype, Google Meet).

Preparation Required

Students will need to complete readings for foundational knowledge about narrative approaches to career development. Students will need to complete the required readings on constructivist approaches to career counseling.

Estimated Time for Delivery of Lesson

Two 3-hour class periods or four 1.5-hour class periods.

Structure and Audience

The lesson can be delivered synchronously to graduate students in a counselor education program using in-person or virtual environments. The instructor may choose an asynchronous approach by recording a narrated PowerPoint presentation.

Lesson Content and Instructional Strategies

Part A: The following will be delivered during the class sessions:

1. Review historical perspective on career counseling from advice-giving to matching the person to a job, to life stages, to a subjective narrative of meanings and adaptability.
2. Student exercise: early recollections, life story chapters
3. Introduce the five life roles: relating, learning, working, pleasuring, valuing
4. Student exercise: life roles circles, current and at a future point (e.g., finishing graduate school)
5. Formulate assessments as qualitative tools: demonstrate card sorts for interests, abilities, values, and Holland typology as (a) like me and not like me and (b) across life roles
6. Student exercise: Draw the Holland Hexagon on a sheet of paper and label the corners R-I-A-S-E-C (realistic, investigative, artistic, social, enterprising, and conventional). Think about going to a party and the people in each corner that reflect the respective

"type," number three corners as your "preferred" types of people, and put an "X" in the corner most not like you. Write examples on the paper in the three corners of what you do that reflect this preference and examples of what you don't like that reflect your "X" corner.

7. Present the storied approach (Brott, 2001) as life chapters and how one's interests, abilities, values, and preferences (i.e., Holland typology) have been experienced. During the presentation, students will draw a personal lifeline and elaborate on one life chapter using their early recollections, preferences, and how their interests, abilities, and values have manifested.
8. Assignment: Students are to create a personal narrative of "finding a life" using the storied approach life chapters across the five life roles listed above that highlight preferences discussed (i.e., typology, interests, abilities, values).

Part B: The following will be delivered during the class sessions:

1. Review guidelines for providing distance professional services. Brainstorm ways to engage clients with virtual qualitative assessments, such as lifeline, life roles circles, Holland typology, and O*NET assessments.
2. Student exercise: Assign student pairs to one qualitative assessment to create an example of delivering the assessment as a video-based synchronous interaction between counselor and client.
3. Demonstrate the qualitative assessment with the student pair outside the classroom and by delivering the assessment to the classroom.
4. Assess the "glows" (strengths) and "grows" (challenges) of providing qualitative assessments through a distance format.

Assessment of Objectives

1. Student submits completed lifeline, life roles circles, and Holland typology "party."
2. Student submits personal narrative of "finding a life" using the storied approach life chapters across the five life roles that highlight preferences (i.e., typology; interests, abilities, values).
3. Student pair demonstrates qualitative assessment using video-based interaction.

4. Students actively participate in assessing the "glows and grows" of providing qualitative assessments through a distance format.

References

Brott, P. E. (2001). The storied approach: A postmodern perspective for career counseling. *Career Development Quarterly, 49*, 301–313. https://doi.org/10.1002/j.2161-0045.2001.tb00958.x

Brott, P. E. (2017). The storied approach. In M. McMahon (Eds.), *Career counselling: Constructivist approaches* (2nd ed.; pp. 93–103). New York: Routledge.

Sample Lesson: Online Career Counseling Approaches to Enhance Career Decision-making

Cameka Hazel, EdD, MHC-LP
New York Institute of Technology
Claudette Brown-Smythe, PhD, LMHC, ACS, NCC, CRC
SUNY Brockport

Lesson Objectives

1) Students will learn how to select appropriate online career assessments and evaluation tools (e.g., choosing cultural, age, and cognitive developmentally appropriate assessments);
2) Students will explore online career information websites to meet the client's needs; and
3) Students will develop an awareness of and utilize career and job marketing social media platforms and digital spaces in tele-career counseling (e.g., LinkedIn, job interviews).

2024 CACREP Standards

Section 3.D (Career Development), Standards 3.D.3 (Processes for identifying and using career, avocational, educational, occupational and labor market information resources, technology, and information systems), 3.D.5 (Strategies for assessing abilities, interests, values, personality and other factors that contribute to career development), and 3.D.6 (Career development program planning, organization, implementation, administration, and evaluation).

Materials and/or Technology Required

Computer, internet access, Zoom/Teams, or other videoconference platform account.

Estimated Time Required for Lesson Delivery

Approximately 3 hours.

Structure and Audience for Lesson

This lesson is structured so that it can be delivered in all formats for counselors in training.

Lesson Content

Career Assessments: The lesson is about selecting appropriate online career assessments and evaluation tools (e.g., choosing cultural, age, and cognitive developmentally appropriate assessments). Career assessments are used to help individuals identify their career goals and interests. The assessments are important because they allow individuals to make well-informed decisions regarding their career interests (Curry et al., 2021). Career assessments that are trait-and-factor approach focused include exploration and learning of self, collecting information on the different careers and the world of work, and using this information to inform career decision-making (e.g., the Holland career key). The results obtained from the administering of career assessments could provide individuals with insights on the careers that are a match for their personality and skills and those that are not, and insights on colleges, universities, and or technical/trade schools that could corroborate with their interests (Curry et al., 2021).

Selecting online career assessments

- These should be reliable and valid. Reliability measures the consistency of the online career assessment tool to measure the constructs. Validity shows how accurate the online assessment is in terms of measuring what it was created to measure (Levin, 2020).
- The CITs should be aware of the normed group. This means the individuals piloting the online assessment tool they are using and the group that additional research was done on to show the effectiveness of the career assessment tool. Norming

information allows the counselor to select the appropriate and effective instrument.

- The CITs should ensure the online assessment is culturally appropriate for the client. CITs should review assessment information to ensure there are no cultural biases, the language is appropriate, and traditional and nontraditional career information is captured for representation of diverse groups' preferences.
- The CITs should consider the client's age and cognitive developmental level when administering the online career assessments. The client should be able to read, understand, and complete the instrument without difficulty.

Exploring online career information websites and online career assessments

Counselors can utilize career websites as resources to help clients during telehealth career counseling. Many of these websites include career assessments for skills, values, and interest awareness.

- CITs can direct clients to these websites to get information on job trends, how to write resumes and cover letters, employment and training programs available, community services and volunteering opportunities, and salary scales.
- CITs should familiarize themselves with the websites before they direct clients to use them. They should be able to give the clients clear directions to find the information on the websites, as some of these websites could appear overwhelming to read because of the amount of information and website layout.
- The following are examples of websites that counselors can use or direct clients to during telehealth sessions:
    - http://online.onetcenter.org
    - http://www.acinet.org/acinet/
    - https://careercycles.com/narrative-system/
    - https://www.naviance.com/
    - https://www.ncda.org/aws/NCDA/pt/sp/resources
    - https://www.careerzone.ny.gov/views/careerzone/index.jsf

There are also online career assessments specifically for school counselors: Kuder Career Planning System, Discover (published by ACT), Naviance, Explore, Holland, and Career Key.

Using online platforms such as LinkedIn, Facebook, and Zoom/Teams for job interviews is a great way career counselors can help their clients develop and market their career portfolios. Counselors can begin by educating their clients about these platforms and their benefits as we enter the digital age. Websites like LinkedIn and Facebook are great for clients to market their skills and abilities. They can also be used to source jobs and research companies. Virtual spaces such as Zoom and Teams are great for connecting people from all over the world. Many clients might prefer to have interviews done through the traditional format; however, the telehealth counselor needs to work with clients to understand contemporary practices so they can maximize their opportunities.

Instructional Strategies

Administering Formal Career Assessment Online

Step 1: Students will be assigned a "client" to administer an online career assessment.

Step 2: Students will visit one of the websites in the following "Additional Resources" list and select a free online career assessment.

Step 3: Students will create an online telehealth appointment with the client to administer the assessment and create a Zoom/Teams link to conduct the assessment.

Step 4: Students will write and present a 2–4 page report on the assessments chosen and the process and evaluation of the assessments. The report should include the following:

1. Who was your client? Give a meaningful background of what you learned from the intake interview.
2. What online career assessment did you use?
3. What does the online career assessment measure?
4. Has the career assessment been normed on multicultural populations? Why do you need to know?
5. How were you able to help your client give meaning to the online career assessment?
6. What interpretation were you able to give to the online career assessment?
7. Did your client find the assessment helpful in the career development process?

Step 5: Students will present the findings in a large-group discussion.

Assessment of Objectives

Students will be assessed on the objectives based on their ability to respond to the questions given in the report.

Additional Resources

- O*NET Online, http://online.onetcenter.org
- CareerOneStop, http://www.acinet.org/acinet/
- CareerCycles, https://careercycles.com/narrative-system/
- NCDA, https://www.ncda.org/aws/NCDA/pt/sp/resources
- CareerZone, https://www.careerzone.ny.gov/views/careerzone/index.jsf

References

Curry, J. R., & Milsom, A. (2021). *Career and college readiness counseling in P-12 schools*. Springer Publishing Company.

Levin, N., Braunstein-Bercovitz, H., Lipshits-Braziler, Y., Gati, I., & Rossier, J. (2020). Testing the structure of the Career Decision-Making Difficulties Questionnaire across country, gender, age, and decision status. *Journal of Vocational Behavior, 116*(Part A), Article 103â365. https://doi.org/10.1016/j.jvb.2019.103365

7

Counseling Practice and Relationships

The practice of telemental health (TMH) counseling has grown significantly over the past few years. Instructors prepare counselors-in-training (CITs) to practice counseling in the field, including face-to-face (F2F) and TMH counseling. CITs need to understand the unique dynamics of TMH counseling and how it varies from F2F interactions. There is a great deal of content to be addressed in the practice of TMH, such as safety and security measures, confidentiality, virtual rapport building, and online communication, as well as variations for TMH modalities, including video, phone, email, and chat services. Instructors who do not have prior training or experience in TMH are encouraged to pursue the training options and suggested readings from Chapter 1.

Key Concepts

CACREP Standards

In line with Section 3.E of the CACREP 2024 Standards, "Counseling Practice and Relationships," master's programs teach content via different courses, typically titled "Counseling Skills," "Counseling Techniques," "Counseling Theories," and "Pre-Practicum." Regardless of the course title, these standards represent the practice of counseling and building counseling relationships, which include TMH counseling and online relationships. In addition, the use of technology is included in this section of the CACREP standards, specifically in Standard 3.E.5, which specifies the program requirement to provide instruction on the application of technology in counseling. Table 7.1 provides examples of how TMH can be infused into counseling practice and relationship instruction. If these concepts are unfamiliar to the instructor, they should review the training and reading materials suggested in Chapter 1.

Table 7.1

CACREP Standards, Section 3.E (Counseling Practice and Relationships) and Suggested TMH Content

CACREP Standards (2024)	Suggested TMH Content
3.E.1. Theories and models of counseling, including relevance to clients from diverse cultural backgrounds.	Examining theories and models from a TMH lens; examine the debate as to whether TMH is a therapeutic intervention in and of itself (Barker & Barker, 2022).
3.E.2. Critical thinking and reasoning strategies for clinical judgment in the counseling process.	Screening clients for TMH and determining if TMH is appropriate for client/student cases (Luxton et al., 2023).
3.E.3. Case conceptualization skills using a variety of models and approaches.	Including technology skills and access in case conceptualization training.
3.E.4. Consultation models and strategies.	Capacity for TMH to support consultation, e.g., other medical providers, collaterals.
3.E.5. Application of technology related to counseling.	Instruction on the practice of TMH counseling, digital record keeping, encryption of software systems, and all uses of technology in counseling practice (e.g., counseling apps).
3.E.6. Ethical and legal issues relevant to establishing and maintaining counseling relationships across service delivery modalities.	Verifying identity and confirming confidential location. Issues of security, encryption, client and counselor competence, etc. (see Chapter 3).

CACREP Standards (2024)	Suggested TMH Content
3.E.7. Culturally sustaining and responsive strategies for establishing and maintaining counseling relationships across service delivery modalities.	Issues of access and opportunity to connect to culturally diverse providers (see Chapter 4).
3.E.8. Counselor characteristics, behaviors, and strategies that facilitate effective counseling relationships.	Skills needed to develop rapport in TMH settings and variations for modalities to create trust and safety (Gluek, 2013).
3.E.9. Interviewing, attending, and listening skills in the counseling process.	Using counseling skills via TMH in various modalities (e.g., phone, video, text; Robertson, 2021).
3.E.10. Counseling strategies and techniques used to facilitate the client change process.	Challenges in digital communication, e.g., verbal and nonverbal communication, technology lags, observation/sensory limits, use of **emojis/emoticons,** and **text-talk**.
3.E.11. Strategies for adapting and accommodating the counseling process to client culture, context, abilities, and preferences.	Using accessible software (see Chapter 14); awareness of cultural context (see Chapter 4).
3.E.12. Goal consensus and collaborative decision-making in the counseling process.	Screen sharing technology for collaborative treatment planning and concurrent documentation.
3.E.13. Developmentally relevant and culturally sustaining counseling treatment or intervention plans.	Ensuring that TMH is appropriate for the developmental stage (see Chapter 5) and culture (see Chapter 4).
3.E.14. Development of measurable outcomes for clients.	Tracking client outcomes in apps; **wearable technology**/biofeedback: **electronic medical records (EMR)** and digital treatment planning; safety planning apps.
3.E.15. Evidence-based counseling strategies and techniques for prevention and intervention.	Examining TMH evidence-based research and its appropriate use for various age groups and clinical foci, much of which focuses on cognitive behavioral therapy (CBT) and/or **iCBT** (internet-based CBT)

CACREP Standards (2024)	Suggested TMH Content
3.E.16. Record-keeping and documentation skills.	Discussion of online documentation security, encryption, and turnkey platforms, e.g., third-party data security; EMR data security; Business Associate Agreements.
3.E.17. Principles and strategies of caseload management and the referral process to promote independence, optimal wellness, empowerment, and engagement with community resources.	Referral process for clients/students for whom TMH is not appropriate or ineffective (see ACA & NBCC Codes of Ethics).
3.E.18. Classification, effects, and indications of commonly prescribed psychopharmacological medications.	Reputable online information sources for information on pharmaceutical medication and other substances (e.g., illegal drugs).
3.E.19. Suicide prevention and response models and strategies.	Emergency management and duty to warn when engaging in TMH. Safety plan apps.
3.E.20. Crisis intervention, trauma-informed, community-based, and disaster mental health strategies.	Emergency management and duty to warn when engaging in TMH; use of the #988 Suicide and Crisis Lifeline, community hotlines, text lines, and other services.
3.E.21 Processes for developing a personal model of counseling grounded in theory and research.	Self-assessment to determine if TMH is appropriate for the counselor and their client base.

Emergency Situations

Emergencies arise in counseling, whether during F2F or TMH counseling. One example includes a client expressing the intent to harm themselves or someone else during a counseling session. Other examples include a medical emergency or a mental health emergency that occurs during a session. The ACA and NBCC Codes of Ethics specify the need for counselors to collect emergency response information and determine policies and procedures for emergencies. The remote location of clients during TMH counseling requires additional action on the part of the counselor. In addition to collecting emergency contact information and preferences during intake, the counselor must also collect information on the nearest medical emergency center, particularly if they are unfamiliar with the client's surrounding area. Best practices dictate that the counselor verifies the client's physical location at the beginning of each session. Since TMH allows clients to be mobile, clients must understand the expectation that they stay at the designated location for the duration of the session. Should emergency personnel be needed, the counselor can demonstrate that they collected the client's location at the start of the session.

Challenges in Online Communication

Videoconferencing is regularly used in TMH counseling. During a videoconference, eye contact can appear skewed, and it may appear that the counselor is not making eye contact with the client. The counselor can adjust the camera to create a more direct angle (Grondin et al., 2021; Grondin et al., 2022). Eye-contact correction software is emerging that fully integrates with video platforms. Through the use of **artificial intelligence** (AI), these programs appear to slowly correct the speaker's gaze to have them look directly at the camera, even when engaging in significant off-screen activity such as reading a teleprompter (Ghosh, 2020). AI can simulate other counselor behaviors, such as head nodding and facial expressions (Choi et al., 2024).

TMH can experience delays due to slow **bandwidth**, frozen video images, or poor mobile reception. Counselors discuss the potential for communication delays with clients and intentionally address silence when it occurs so all parties know that communication is not lost. TMH limits observation and sensory skills that can be utilized in the session. Research shows that clients prefer a "close-up" image of a counselor instead of a farther, zoomed-out, full-body image (Grondin et al., 2021). Telephone sessions do not allow counselors to see the client. In phone sessions, facial expressions are missing, as are the emotions displayed on one's face. During phone sessions, counselors should probe for emotional, physical, and bodily responses. Nonverbal cues can also include the client's appearance, gait, odor, and hygiene, which are missing from phone and videoconferencing sessions. These observations may be a critical component of an assessment, diagnosis, or mental status exam for people with addiction and mental health disorders.

Counseling via email, text, chat, or messaging can create new challenges. One common concern is the privacy and security of written communications since email, text, chat, or messaging can create a written transcript of the dialogue between counselors and clients. Counselors should explain security precautions being taken, such as encrypted devices, to clients. Even still, clients may be comfortable communicating verbally but not comfortable communicating in writing. For example, people speaking their non-native language may be comfortable speaking but less comfortable writing in a non-native language. Counselors using text and messaging apps must understand **text-type** communication, which uses abbreviations, acronyms, and **emojis** to communicate. Chat and text messaging are not a "real-time" interaction. Messages sent may remain unread for long periods of time. Because counselors and clients compose messages before sending, they have more time to think, rewrite, and craft the message to clearly convey their intended thoughts. This causes concern that messages may be less genuine. Conversely, some clients may send off messages via text or email with little thought and planning. Some may struggle to communicate emotion in writing. Counselors may need to probe directly for emotion or encourage clients to use emoticons to reflect emotion. How often asynchronous messages will be reviewed and responded to is explicitly outlined in informed consent documents.

Teaching Techniques

Instructors can introduce the practice of TMH in a variety of ways. Below is a list of suggested strategies that might reinforce or supplement the CITs' understanding of TMH professional practice. These strategies utilize andragogical principles, including self-motivated learning, using prior experiences, recognizing a need for information, and immediately applying learning in a real-world context (Knowles, 1975).

1. *TMH Logistics.* TMH requires thought and planning, regardless of the modality used. Have CITs discuss and document what steps and precautions they would need to take before engaging in TMH practice via phone, video, email, or chat. Consider both physical and technological issues. Robertson (2021) contains a checklist for preparing for TMH practice in the appendix, which may be helpful for this activity.
2. *Screening for TMH.* Using TMH requires that the client be appropriate for TMH services, including developmentally, clinically, and technologically. CITs can discuss and document what screening questions/information they would need to gather from a client before engaging in TMH practice, including referral sources and emergency contacts. The instructor can create fictional cases in which CITs can practice screening.

3. *Verifying Identity for TMH.* TMH requires that counselors verify the identity of their clients, whether practicing via video, phone, email, or chat. Have CITs role-play verifying identity with clients in each modality.
4. *Practice TMH Skills via Video.* CITs can practice mock TMH sessions via video with their peers using the tools outlined in Chapter 2. CITs can share the strengths and challenges of TMH in this modality.
5. *Practice TMH Skills via Phone.* CITs can practice mock TMH sessions via phone with their peers using the tools outlined in Chapter 2. Have CITs share the strengths and challenges of TMH in this modality.
6. *Practice TMH Skills via Email.* CITs can provide mock TMH sessions via email with their peers using the tools outlined in Chapter 2. Be aware of email precautions and transcripts. Have CITs share the strengths and challenges of TMH in this modality.
7. *Practice TMH Skills via Chat/Messaging.* CITs can provide mock TMH sessions via chat/messaging with their peers using the tools outlined in Chapter 2. Be aware of chat/messaging precautions and transcripts. CITs can share the strengths and challenges of TMH in this modality.
8. *Reflecting Emotion via Multiple Modalities.* From the mock sessions suggested above, CITs should attempt to reflect emotion in each modality. Have CITs discuss the strengths and challenges of reflecting emotion in each modality.
9. *Assessing Lethality via Multiple Modalities.* Assessing the lethality of the client or others is a critical part of a counselor's job. CITs can role-play assessing lethality in multiple modalities and process how they felt doing so in each setting, including time-delayed modalities, such as chat or email.
10. *Contacting Emergency Contacts via TMH.* At times, counselors need to notify an emergency contact, whether it be a client's appointed emergency contact or local officials. Have CITs discuss the steps and strategies needed in preparation for these instances. CITs can role-play having to contact an emergency contact (or dispatching emergency services) via multiple modalities while keeping the client engaged.

Sample Lesson:
Counseling Skills Practice in Multiple TMH Modalities

Tyce Nadrich, PhD, LMHC, NCC, ACS
Mercer University

Lesson Objective(s)

At the end of this lesson, students will have

1) practiced their learned counseling skills in four counseling modalities, including in-person, video, phone, and text message/ chat,
2) examined their strengths and challenges in each modality, and
3) received feedback on their counseling skills in each modality.

2024 CACREP Standards

Section 3.E (Counseling Practice and Relationships), Standards 3.E.5 (Application of technology related to counseling), and 3.E.9 (Interviewing, attending, and listening skills in the counseling process).

Materials and/or Technology Required

1) Students need access to a videoconferencing system with audio, video, and chat capabilities, as well as recording and the option to download videos.
2) A learning management system (LMS) for students to submit recordings.
3) Students may be required to obtain malpractice insurance before engaging in mock sessions (see accreditation, state, and program or university guidelines).

Preparation Required

Prior instruction on counseling skills, such as the *Microskills Hierarchy* (Ivey et al., 2018), as well as the practice of TMH and distance counseling in various modalities (Robertson, 2021).

Estimated Time Required for Lesson Delivery

This activity is conducted via five weekly assignments. The weekly assignments should take the student approximately 1 hour (a 20-minute video and a 40-minute reflection) per week. The instructor will process student reflections following the assignment for approximately 15–30 minutes each week.

Structure and Audience for Lesson

This activity is designed for master's students in counseling programs learning counseling skills. The lesson may be adapted for in-person, online synchronous, and online asynchronous instruction.

Lesson Content and Instructional Strategies

Many counseling programs assess counseling skills by having students engage in mock counseling sessions with peers. That model is used for this lesson, but the modality of the mock sessions varies throughout the five sessions, while the client/counselor pair remains the same.

1. Students are paired with a partner to practice the counseling skills they have been learning in class, such as the microskills hierarchy or other models of counseling skills.
2. Students are assigned weekly mock counseling sessions, where each student will play both the counselor and the client (e.g., every student will submit five recordings where they are the counselor). During these recordings, student-clients should be discussing low-level concerns appropriate for a beginning counselor in training (e.g., common stressors, difficulties with adjustment).
3. The first and last counseling sessions are conducted in-person and recorded, modeling best practices of beginning distance therapy in-person when possible.
4. The modalities for the second, third, and fourth sessions are up to the counselor. One session must be conducted with video and audio capability turned on, another must be conducted with audio on and video off, and the final must be conducted using a message/chat feature with video and audio off. All sessions are recorded.
5. After each mock session, the student engages in a reflection and self-assessment activity as assigned by the instructor. Some

instructors utilize process transcripts, while others use reflective journals. However, the reflection and self-assessment activity must include a reflection on the counseling skills used during each session.

6. The video and the reflection are uploaded to the LMS for instructor review and feedback. Feedback is provided to students on their skills for each session.
7. Each week, following the submission of the recording and reflection of the first four sessions, the instructor leads a group discussion on their use of counseling skills in each modality. Sample questions may include:
    a. What were your strengths and challenges with this session?
    b. How did the modality of the session impact your counseling skills?
    c. How did the modality of the session impact the client's responses?
    d. What did you learn specifically about using this modality?
    e. How likely are you to use this modality with future clients/ students?
    f. What did you learn, or what would you do differently, if you used this modality again?

Following the final session, the instructor leads a discussion comparing all modalities. Some sample questions may include: 1) Compare and contrast all modalities. 2) What were the strengths and benefits of each? 3) Which modality do you feel would be positive or negative with specific populations? Why or why not? 4) What final thoughts do you have about being required to use all modalities during this class?

Assessment of Objectives

The instructor provides feedback on the student's counseling skills by reviewing each session's recordings and reflections. Lesson objectives can also be assessed via the classroom discussion and the students' response to the activity.

Possible Modification for Advanced Counseling Skills

For instructors seeking to incorporate this lesson toward the end of a counseling skills class, an advanced skills class, a course specifically designed for TMH counseling, or any other advanced counseling course or elective, the following option is suggested:

- Broaching across modalities: In this modification, each student-client will be provided with a script from the course instructor that will require broaching. The references below will help inform students about the concept and specific methods. Students will be required to broach at least once in each modality (in person, video and audio, audio only, and text only). Thereafter, in addition to the reflection content highlighted previously, students will also reflect on how broaching approaches varied across modalities.
    - Day-Vines, N. L., Wood, S., Grothaus, T., Craigen, L., Holman, A., Dotson-Blake, K., & Douglass, M. (2007). *Broaching the subjects of race, ethnicity, and culture during the counseling process. 85*(4), 401–409. https://doi.org/10.1002/j.1556-6678.2007.tb00608.x
    - Day-Vines, N. L., Booker, A. B., Steen, S., & Arnold, K. M. (2018). Getting comfortable with discomfort: Preparing counselor trainees to broach racial, ethnic, and cultural factors with clients during counseling. *International Journal for the Advancement of Counselling,* 40, 89–104. https://doi.org/10.1007/s10447-017-9308-9

References

Ivey, A. E., Ivey, M .B., & Zalaquett, C. P. (2018). *Intentional interviewing and counseling: Facilitating client development in a multicultural society* (9th ed.). Brooks/Cole.

Robertson, H. C. (2021). *Telemental health and distance counseling: A counselor's guide to decisions, resources, and practice.* Springer Publishing Company.

Sample Lesson:
The Application of Smartphone Apps to Counseling Practice

Ming-hui Li, EdD, LMHC, LPC
St. John's University

Lesson Objectives

1) To learn about the benefits and limitations of using apps in counseling practice, and
2) To learn about the process of developing a counseling approach that integrates apps with traditional counseling theories.

2024 CACREP Standards

Section 3.E (Counseling Practice and Relationships), Standards 3.E.1 (Theories and models of counseling), and 3.E.5 (Application of technology related to counseling).

Materials and/or Technology Required

Students download a counseling-related app to their mobile phones.

Preparation Required

1) Students complete an assignment that uses an integrative approach (in this case, two different counseling theories) to counsel a client in a case example;
2) Students are expected to practice the counseling app they download and become familiar with its functions.

Estimated Time Required for Lesson Delivery

One hour.

Structure and Audience for Lessons

The lesson can be conducted online synchronously or in person. The audience is graduate students taking a "Counseling Theories" or similar course.

Lesson Content and Instructional Strategies

1. *Introduction:* Begin by introducing the topic of using apps in counseling and explaining the purpose of the lesson, which is to introduce the idea of integrating apps with counseling approaches in the counseling process. Discuss the benefits and limitations of this integrative approach to counseling.
2. *Presentation #1:* Provide an overview of the different types of apps that are available for counseling, such as mood-tracking apps, mindfulness apps, and cognitive behavioral therapy (CBT) apps. Next, students conduct presentations to introduce the apps that they downloaded to their mobile phones. Then, students presented their assignment of using an integrative approach (in this case, two counseling theories) to counsel a client in a case example.
3. *Group discussion:* Divide the class into small groups and discuss the app they downloaded onto their mobile phone and their thoughts and experiences with using apps in counseling. Encourage open and honest dialogue and facilitate the discussion as needed.
4. *Presentation #2:* The instructor provides the class with information about the benefits and risks of applying smartphone apps to counseling practice. The potential benefits include increased accessibility to counseling, convenience, flexibility in scheduling appointments, and the ability to reach underserved populations. The risks include security and confidentiality concerns, lack of regulation and oversight, inadequate training and competence of app providers, potential for misuse and harm, difficulty in building rapport and a therapeutic relationship, and insufficient empirical support for efficacy.
5. *Case study:* Two students play a video of a mock counseling session in which two counseling approaches are integrated (based on their completed assignment mentioned in procedure # 2 in this section).
6. *Discussion:* The class discusses possible ways to incorporate apps into the case example. Encourage students to consider the potential benefits and risks of using the app in this context.

Conclusion: Summarize the lesson's key points and encourage the class to consider how they might incorporate apps and traditional counseling approaches into their counseling practice. Encourage students to continue exploring the use of apps in counseling and to stay up to date on the latest research and resources.

Assessment of Objectives

*(Correct answer indicated by the asterisk *)*

1) Which of the following is not a benefit of applying mobile apps to counseling practice?
    a. increased flexibility in scheduling appointments
    b. increased accessibility to counseling
    c. the ability to reach underserved populations
    d. enhanced therapeutic relationship *
2) Which of the following is not a limitation of applying mobile apps to counseling practice?
    a. security and confidentiality concerns
    b. difficult to access *
    c. potential for misuse and harm
    d. insufficient empirical support for efficacy
3) Briefly describe one possible way to integrate an app with traditional counseling approaches to counsel the client in the case example mentioned in this lesson.

References

Corey, G. (2017). *Theory and Practice of Counseling and Psychotherapy* (10th ed.). Cengage Learning.

Goss, S., Anthony, K., Stretch, L. S., Nagel, D. M. (2016). *Technology in Mental Health: Application in Practice, Supervision and Training* (2nd ed.). Thomas.

Lui, J. H. L., Marcus, D. K., & Barry, C. T. (2017). Evidence-based apps? A review of mental health mobile applications in a psychotherapy context. *Professional Psychology: Research and Practice, 48*(3), 199–210. http://doi.org/10.1037/pro0000122

Robertson, H. (2021). *Telemental health and distance counseling: A counselor's guide to decisions, resources, and practice*. Springer.

8

Group Work and Group Counseling

Telemental health (TMH) counseling can be delivered individually as well as in groups. Counselors-in-training (CITs) may be required to deliver TMH counseling in group settings. Instructors training counselors in the delivery of TMH groups can begin by encouraging CITs to define the type of group they are running. The Association for Specialists in Group Work (ASGW) specifies that different groups have different scopes of practice and, as such, may be held to different standards under the law (ASGW, 2021). Based on licensing laws and the possibility of conducting TMH groups across state lines, TMH counselors need to define the type of group they are administering and adhere to the legal and ethical guidelines of the identified group type.

ASGW publishes the *Guiding Principles for Group Work*, a "principled framework" where group workers can find "a contemporary integration of ethical practice, contextual perspectives, and organizational values with the intent to guide group scholars and practitioners" (ASGW, 2021, p. 1). The document supplements the ACA Code of Ethics in that "nothing in this document shall be construed to supplant that code" (ASGW, 2021, p.3). While this document serves as a guide for group counseling, instructors should note that the ethical codes of other organizations also have content pertaining to group work, including ACA (Section

A.9, Group Work), ASCA (Section A.7, Group Work), AMHCA (Sections I.B.3.c and I.B.3.d), NCDA (Section A.8, Group Work), as well as the Commission on Rehabilitation Counselor Certification (CRCC, 2022; Section A.6 Group Work), and NAADAC, the Association for Addiction Professionals (2021; Standard I-14, Group). Instructors and CITs should consider all ethical codes and contexts in which the practice of TMH group work may be applied.

Key Concepts

CACREP Standards

Section 3.F of the CACREP 2024 Standards (Group Counseling and Group Work) is a core curricular area practiced in multiple specializations, as indicated by the ethical codes above. It is also one of the few areas of the CACREP standards that includes technology, specifically Standard 3.F.6. Table 8.1 provides examples of how TMH can be infused into group counseling courses. If these concepts are unfamiliar to the instructor, they should review the training and reading materials suggested in Chapter 1.

Table 8.1

CACREP Section 3.F (Group Counseling and Group Work) and Suggested TMH Content

CACREP Standards (2024)	Suggested TMH Content
3.F.1. Theoretical foundations of group counseling and group work.	Exploration of how group counseling can be adapted for and impacted by TMH delivery.
3.F.2. Dynamics associated with group process and development.	The dynamics of group process in a virtual setting, accounting for different modalities of connecting to the group (e.g., video, phone).
3.F.3. Therapeutic factors of group work and how they contribute to group effectiveness.	Capacity of TMH groups to promote universality and shared experience among clients from remote locations (Weiss et al., 2018).
3.F.4. Characteristics and functions of effective group leaders.	Skills to lead TMH groups, including client engagement and managing talk time virtually (Guth et al., 2020; Robertson, 2021).

CACREP Standards (2024)	Suggested TMH Content
3.F.5. Approaches to group formation, including recruiting, screening, and selecting members.	Setting expectations for online groups (Guth et al., 2020; Hunter & Rewa, 2020).
3.F.6. Application of technology related to group counseling and group work.	Managing groups online (Whittingham & Martin, 2020); technological safety and security (see Chapter 3).
3.F.7. Types of groups, settings, and other considerations that affect conducting groups.	Legal and ethical practices of leading different group types in compliance with licensing requirements.
3.F.8. Culturally sustaining and developmentally responsive strategies for designing and facilitating groups.	Online group barriers to establishing trust (Kozlowski & Holmes, 2014, 2017).
3.F.9. Ethical and legal considerations relative to the delivery of group counseling and group work across service delivery modalities.	ASGW Standards (2021), ACA (2014), National Board for Certified Counselors (NBCC; 2023), and other codes, re: group work and TMH practice; state statutes; risks of online open groups.
3.F.10. Direct experiences in which counseling students participate as group members in a small group activity, approved by the program, for a minimum of 10 clock hours over the course of one academic term.	Students should be exposed to online groups as facilitators, group members, or observers to identify group content and group process as a component of their 10 hours of group counseling training.

Facilitating Online Groups

The Community Technical Assistance Center of New York (CTACNY) recommends setting aside the first session of a group meeting to review the technology with group members (2020). To mitigate safety concerns, they recommend collecting crisis contact information, confirming locations during sessions, and determining barriers to emergency resources for group members, such as geographic distance from emergency services.

ASGW published a document titled *Ten Tips for the Facilitation of Virtual Groups* (Guth et al., 2020), which is helpful for both instructors and CITs alike. The document, drawn from recent literature, provides guidelines for TMH group facilitation. This document begins with selecting the best technology for the group and setting the stage for group work, including testing the technology, following ethical guidelines, and preparing for TMH groups. "Setting the stage" requires the group leader to minimize multitasking and distractions while encouraging the group members to do the same. This may include logging out of other applications, such as email, and putting away mobile phones. Hunter and Rewa (2020) recommend setting expectations before the group and naming distractions at the beginning of the group through statements such as "Prepare to be fully present" or asking, "Do you need to remove a pet from the room or put away a mobile device?" (Hunter & Rewa, 2020, p. 8). CITs need to model being fully present as they facilitate online groups.

Engaging Online Group Members

There are many types of members who join online groups. CITs need strategies to manage different behaviors that could occur in groups. These may include unwanted interruptions during live synchronous groups (e.g., **zoom bombers**) and different levels of participation in both synchronous and asynchronous groups, such as posters and **lurkers** (Boniel-Nissim, 2016) in online asynchronous groups. CITs need to learn to engage group members effectively during online group administration.

Trust and rapport are cornerstones of the counseling relationship. Based on the larger number of members, trust could be more challenging to establish in group counseling than face-to-face counseling (F2F). TMH groups can create additional barriers to establishing trust (Kozlowski & Holmes, 2014, 2017). CITs can enhance trust by modeling and naming ethical practices they are engaging in to establish trust. These practices include using their headphones and cameras to scan the room so members see they are in a confidential space. It includes establishing and reinforcing ground rules. Rapport is enhanced when group leaders use members' names and encourage members to dialogue with one another. It is enhanced by noticing a member's emotional state and reflecting on that observation. These rapport-building skills can be more challenging in an online setting. CITs must continually work on these skills to create an effective online group dynamic.

Online group facilitators also engage online group members by using activities and demonstrating energy and attentiveness toward the group dynamics. This may include having members engage in an intentional activity instead of simply listening. For example, members could write a response in the chat or select an emoji that portrays their mood. Online group facilitators can be creative by using visual displays, audio, or video to engage the group. Sometimes, even the most creative attempts will fall flat. Other times, the group facilitator will have a plan, only for another event, such as a client crisis or world event, to occur and require the alteration of that plan. As with F2F groups, online group facilitators need to display flexibility and a willingness to adapt to the group's needs. Limiting the number of people in the group will help keep members engaged, as large numbers make it harder for all members to participate and easier for members to disengage (Choudhuri, 2020). CITs need to practice engaging members in an online group if they have not done so in the past.

Teaching Techniques

Instructors can introduce group TMH counseling practice in a variety of ways. Below is a list of suggested strategies that might reinforce or supplement CITs' understanding of TMH group counseling. These strategies utilize andragogical principles, including self-motivated learning, using prior experiences, recognizing a need for information, and immediately applying learning in a real-world context (Knowles, 1975).

1. *Observing Open Online Groups.* Some self-help organizations (e.g., Alcoholics Anonymous, Narcotics Anonymous, Overeaters Anonymous) host online open groups in multiple formats (e.g., video, phone, discussion boards). These are support groups and not counseling groups, and CITs should be respectful observers in an open group to experience online group dynamics. CITs need to remember that the groups must be open, group content should be confidential, and they must respect the established group norms and guidelines (including "no visitors," should that occur).
2. *Participating in Online Groups.* Master's students in CACREP programs must participate in at least 10 hours of small-group counseling activities. CITs can experience a portion of their hours, or additional hours, in a TMH format and explore how group processes and dynamics may vary in both TMH and face-to-face (F2F) group settings.
3. *Engaging Online Unengaged Clients.* CITs can role-play facilitating an online group with peers (using the technological tools discussed in Chapter 2). The instructor can privately message some students to be disengaged while the leader attempts to engage those group members. CITs can process the experience both as leaders and group members at the conclusion of the role-play.

Consider various modalities like video, phone, and discussion board groups.

4. *Calming Online Irate Clients.* CITs can role-play facilitating an online group with peers. The instructor can privately message some students to play an irate group member who appears to argue with another member while the leader attempts to focus the group. CITs process the experience both as leaders and group members at the conclusion of the role-play. Consider various modalities like video, phone, and discussion board groups.
5. *Talk About It: Late Arrivals.* Many F2F groups have policies about late arrivals. CITs should discuss how they would handle late arrivals for online groups, including various modalities like phone and video. CITs should consider the following: What policies might need to be developed or enforced to address these issues? Does the reason for the lateness matter?
6. *Talk About It: Cameras Off.* Many online video groups have policies about cameras being on during group sessions. What are the pros and cons of that type of policy? CITs can explore how they might address clients with their cameras off, assuming they have the audio, video, and chat features available. Have CITs explore the pros and cons of addressing the issue in multiple ways and how they'd address a member who does not comply. What would they do if the camera didn't work?
7. *Talk About It: Disrespecting Ground Rules.* Group norms or ground rules help guide group work and help create a safe and respectful group for all. Have CITs explore how they might address/respond to a group member disrespecting group rules. Some examples include being late, having cameras off, having people in the background (not in a confidential space), being in a public place, not being dressed appropriately for a group session, being visibly distracted (on the phone, talking to someone else), or using disparaging, racist, or disrespectful language toward another member.
8. *The Case of Disconnection.* Here is an example case scenario: You are running a TMH group, and Member A suddenly drops off the video. You continue the group, and since your email and phone are off, you don't notice any other messages. Member B interrupts the person speaking to tell you that Member A is trying to reach you via email. You explain that you are not checking your email currently. Member B has their mobile phone in their hand and

appears to be texting but then stops and appears to be typing on a keyboard. While the other group member continues to talk, you get a private message from Member B that Member A is texting them and would like Member B to put them on speaker phone so they can rejoin the group. How do you proceed?

9. *Brainstorming for Engaging Activities.* One of the benefits of online groups is that the leader and group members can share media and resources that may be beneficial or related to the group. Have CITs brainstorm different activities for using online technology during group that would help keep members engaged. Consider ways group members might participate beyond watching or listening to content.
10. *Practicing Our Focus.* We are a multitasking society and often have multiple applications simultaneously running on phones and laptops. Instructors can engage CITs in a voluntary anonymous activity where they record how many programs they have open on their devices. For example, during in-person or synchronous classes, instructors can use an anonymous poll for students to record the number of programs open. Instructors can challenge CITs to narrow their focus during class and offer random follow-up polls to assess their progress. Instructors should remind CITs that TMH groups require focus and complete attention.

Sample Lesson: Developing Informed Consent for Online Groups Using ChatGPT

Nouna Jalilzadeh, PhD, LMHC, NCC
St. John's University

Lesson Objective

The purpose of this lesson is to encourage students to embrace the use of technology, ethically and responsibly, in the counseling process. At the conclusion of this lesson, students will have examined the ACA Code of Ethics and the ASGW Guiding Principles for essential elements of informed consent documents, demonstrated and identified ethical considerations and implications of utilizing artificial intelligence, and will draft informed consent documents using ChatGPT or other artificial intelligence (AI) platforms.

2024 CACREP Standards

Standards 3.F.6 (Application of technology related to group counseling and group work) and 3.F.9 (Ethical and legal considerations relative to the delivery of group counseling and group work across service delivery modalities).

Materials and/or Technology Required

Access to ChatGPT or other AI technology. If the lesson is being delivered in person, students will need to bring laptops or other devices to access ChatGPT or other AI technology. At least half of the students should have an account on ChatGPT or other AI technology platform. Access to samples of informed consent for online groups from 2–3 diverse clientele practices, the ACA Code of Ethics, and the ASGW guiding principles.

Preparation Required

Students need prior instruction on group counseling ethics and online group counseling. Using prior information in this chapter, the ACA Code of Ethics, and the ASGW guiding principles, students need prior training in elements of Informed Consent. Students will also need to have a basic understanding of ChatGPT or other AI technology platforms and their purposes and capabilities.

Estimated Time Required for Lesson Delivery

Prior instruction time may vary. The time for this activity is approximately 60–90 minutes. If delivered online synchronously or asynchronously, students can work independently or in pairs; however, if working independently, each must have access to ChatGPT/AI technology.

Structure and Audience for Lesson

This activity is best used in in-person or online synchronous classroom settings, including master's, doctoral, or professional development training. However, adaptations can be made for online asynchronous learning via learning management systems (LMS) and recorded videos, discussion boards, and video presentations.

Lesson Content and Instructional Strategies

1. The instructor provides instructional content to students on group dynamics, group ethics, online groups, and ethics pertaining to facilitating in-person and online groups.
2. The instructor introduces the role of AI, specifically ChatGPT, and discusses potential benefits, challenges, and ethical considerations of using ChatGPT/AI for therapeutic purposes.
3. The instructor introduces the activity as a way for students to ethically, responsibly, and critically utilize technology in their counseling practice.
4. For this activity, students are asked to use ChatGPT/AI software to write an ethical and accurate informed consent document for an online group.
5. Depending on the number of students, students are encouraged to work in pairs or groups where at least one member can access ChatGPT/AI software.
6. Pairs or groups are asked to choose and focus on an online counseling group type or topic (e.g., emotion regulation, depression, postpartum) and draft a consent form utilizing ChatGPT/AI.
7. Students provide an initial prompt to the ChatGPT/AI software, such as "Write me an informed consent for online (type/topic) group counseling sessions."
8. After receiving their initial response, students use the ACA Code of Ethics and ASGW Guiding Principles, including group work, distance counseling content, and informed consent samples provided earlier, to add follow-up questions and have ChatGPT edit the document. For example, students might add statements such as "add content on facilitating online groups," "edit to include information on technology risks," "add resources and information related to the type of the group," or "add content on emergency contacts."
9. Based on what the software creates, students add elements to their document until they feel they have a solid informed consent that they are satisfied with.
10. After enough time, the instructor brings the group back together for a final discussion/reflection.
11. Each group will present their informed consent subsections and answer the following questions:
    a. How was it for them to use this software in this way?

b. Look at the first informed consent the software gave you and compare it to your final version. What are some of the elements you added along the way?
c. How did you consider your group types and topics when developing your consent?
d. What were some of the areas from the ACA/ASGW codes that you added and why?
e. How satisfied are you with the final product? Is it something you would use with a client? Why or why not?
f. How do you feel about using this technology to support counseling practice? Would you use it for other documentation, such as treatment plans or case notes? Why or why not? What responsibility do we have to the client to inform them of our use of technology, if any?
g. Any other comments about the experience?

Assessment of Objective

Assessment of the lesson objective will be done via the classroom discussion/dialogue and the student's response to the activity. Instructors may also require students to submit their activity (e.g., download a transcript from the AI with multiple variations) as evidence of their engagement. Pairs and groups can also engage in a peer-review process, looking at one another's informed consent documents and providing feedback.

Sample Lesson: Preparing for Online Group Attacks

Qiana Spellman, EdD, Certified School Counselor
St. John's University

Lesson Objective

At the end of this lesson, students will have practiced maintaining a safe and supportive environment while managing online attacks as they facilitate open online groups.

2024 CACREP Standards

Standards 3.F.6 (Application of technology related to group counseling and group work) and 3.F.4 (Characteristics and functions of effective group leaders).

Materials or Technology Required

Technology to facilitate a mock online counseling session, including the capacity for all members to share screens, unmute themselves and use the chat feature.

Preparation Required

Students need prior instruction on group dynamics and group facilitation of online groups, including the potential for online attacks in the group and the facilitator's role in protecting their clients from harm.

Estimated Time Required for Lesson Delivery

While prior instruction time may vary, the time for this activity is approximately 20–30 minutes.

Structure and Audience for Lesson

This activity is designed for online synchronous classroom settings, including master's, doctoral, or professional development training.

- The activity format is fully described to students before its implementation; emphasize that no attacking language or images will be used.
- The instructor will set the stage for this as a practice activity for online attacks while ensuring a safe space for all those involved.
- The instructor should use caution when considering this lesson, based on the group's cohesion, comfort and trust with one another, and professionalism.

Lesson Content and Instructional Strategies

1. The instructor will create an online group session where all members can share their screens, unmute themselves, and use the chat feature.
2. The lesson and its purpose are fully explained to students before the activity begins. If a class member feels the activity may be a trigger, they can be excused from participating.
   a. Before the activity begins, all students will be asked to open a Word document that displays the words to be used if they are assigned the role of attacker. On the Word document, students will type the following exactly as they appear in

quotations: "sexually explicit content," "graphic or violent content," or "mental health trigger content." They can type each phrase in quotations on a separate page. No other words or images should be used beyond those in the quotations above. Students should use plain font and not seek to involve any other emotional responses than the phrases above. Specifically, the student is only writing the words "mental health trigger" and is NOT coming up with or including any examples of what might be considered an actual mental health trigger.

b. It is imperative that the instructor emphasize that for this activity, students will only use these exact words. To avoid creating trauma or a triggering classroom context, students playing the role of the attackers may only use the phrases: "sexually explicit content," "graphic or violent content," or "mental health trigger content." No additional words, phrases, or images will be allowed during this activity.

c. One student will volunteer to be the group facilitator. If the activity is repeated, students will rotate in this role.

d. The instructor will privately assign two students to be the online "attackers." The instructor will privately message the two students that they are the "attackers" for this session and assign them sharing permissions if needed. The attackers will also vary with each facilitator if repeated.

3. The facilitator will be assigned the role of "host" and will begin the session with an ethical opening and a review of the online group rules. They will then engage in a mock session, checking in with members on how their week has been. The online members may be asked to unmute themselves and share verbally or to write their responses in the chat.
4. The attackers will randomly take themselves off mute, use the screen sharing feature, or use the chat feature to display the attacking content. For example, one attacker may come off mute and say "sexually explicit content," while the other member continually types "mental health trigger content" in the chat feature. Or either attacker might suddenly share their screen with the words "graphic or violent content."
5. The facilitator will need to try to navigate the situation by either addressing the behavior, muting the participant, or removing them from the group.

6. The instructor will end the activity after a reasonable amount of time, typically no more than 5–10 minutes.
   a. The instructor will facilitate a group discussion with the class, specifically addressing:
   b. How the group facilitator felt trying to manage the group and the attackers.
   c. How the group members felt during the exercise.
   d. How the attackers felt during the exercise and with the role they were assigned.
   e. Feedback for the group facilitator on how they managed the situation.
   f. Recommendations on how to manage similar situations in the future.
   g. While this was only a simulation, how would you feel if it were an actual attack?
   h. Any other comments and/or questions.
7. If the instructor and the students wish, another facilitator and attackers can be selected for additional practice, repeating items 3–7 above.

Assessment of Objective

Assessment of the lesson objective will be examined via the classroom discussion and the students' responses to the activity. Students may also be asked to reference this activity in a reflective journal of other assignments.

9

Assessment and Diagnostic Processes

The task of conducting assessments varies depending on the counselor's position. In a school setting, assessment for learning disabilities and mental health conditions is often relegated to the school psychologist or external providers. However, school counselors may assess students via formal measures, such as the Conners Rating Scale (Conners, 2022), or informal measures, such as classroom observation or interviews (Whitson, 2017). Addiction counselors regularly use standardized addiction assessments, such as the Alcohol Use Disorders Identification Test (AUDIT; Baber et al., 2001) or the American Society of Addiction Medicine (ASAM) Criteria Assessment Interview (ASAM, 2022), but cannot administer standardized instruments for mental health diagnoses. Mental health counselors conduct assessments of mental health conditions to support a diagnosis, develop treatment plans, and bill insurance. When assessment services are delivered via telemental health (TMH), counselors must adapt their assessment practices to TMH parameters. Instructors need to help counselors-in-training (CITs) understand the unique elements of assessment when engaging in distance practices.

Key Concepts

CACREP Standards

CACREP changed the standard for this core curriculum area from "Assessment and Testing" in the 2016 standards to "Assessment and Diagnostic Processes" in the 2024 version (CACREP, 2016, 2024). This change requires that all counselors, not just mental health counselors, receive training in diagnostic processes. TMH instruction for CITs must include both information on conducting assessments and engaging in diagnostic processes via TMH modalities. Table 9.1 provides examples of how TMH can be infused into assessment and diagnosis training. If these concepts are unfamiliar, the instructor is encouraged to explore the training and reading materials suggested in Chapter 1.

Table 9.1

CACREP Section 3.G (Assessment and Diagnostic Processes) and Suggested TMH Content

CACREP Standards (2024)	Suggested TMH Content
3.G.1. Historical perspectives concerning the nature and meaning of assessment and testing in counseling.	TMH history, beginning with psychiatry and remote assessment of mental health conditions (Breen & Matusitz, 2010).
3.G.2. Basic concepts of standardized and non-standardized testing, norm-referenced and criterion-referenced assessments, and group and individual assessments.	Examining assessment manuals for developing instruments normed for TMH use; guidelines on validation or adaptation to online delivery (Corey & Ben-Porath, 2020; Krach et al., 2020; Pearson, 2021).
3.G.3. Statistical concepts, including scales of measurement, measures of central tendency, indices of variability, shapes and types of distributions, and correlations.	Ability to communicate assessment results to clients, students, and/or parents during online meetings; understanding statistical concepts as necessary for accurate explanations.
3.G.4. Reliability and validity in the use of assessments.	Accessing online information tools to identify reliable and valid measures, e.g., Mental Measurements Yearbook/Tests in Print.

CACREP Standards (2024)	Suggested TMH Content
3.G.5. Culturally sustaining and developmental considerations for selecting, administering, and interpreting assessments, including individual accommodations and environmental modifications.	History of misuse of assessment with cultural and minority groups—same risks via TMH. Selecting culturally appropriate assessments normed for diverse populations and TMH delivery. Benefit of accessing diverse clients and providers (see Chapter 4).
3.G.6. Ethical and legal considerations for selecting, administering, and interpreting assessments.	Evaluation of counseling ethical codes pertaining to assessment and TMH and the Standards for Educational and Psychological Testing (American Educational Research Association [AERA; 2014]).
3.G.7. Use of culturally sustaining and developmentally appropriate assessments for diagnostic and intervention planning purposes.	Using current instruments, normed on diverse populations and for TMH delivery.
3.G.8. Use of assessments in academic/educational, career, personal, and social development.	Review of assessment use in different settings, including identifying instruments for each setting appropriate for TMH delivery.
3.G.9. Use of environmental assessments and systematic behavioral observations.	Challenges of environmental and behavioral observations from a distance; strategies for remote client/student observation.
3.G.10. Use of structured interviewing, symptom checklists, and personality and psychological testing.	*Checklist for Conducting Remote Psychological Testing Proctored via Teleconference* (Corey & Ben-Porath, 2020, p. 202).
3.G.11. Diagnostic processes, including differential diagnosis and the use of current diagnostic classification systems.	Obstacles to assessing and determining a mental health diagnosis via TMH (see Chapter 13).
3.G.12. Procedures to identify substance use, addictions, and co-occurring conditions.	Challenges of limited observation and non-verbal cues (e.g., odor, hygiene) (see Chapter 11).

CACREP Standards (2024)	Suggested TMH Content
3.G.13. Procedures for assessing and responding to risk of aggression or danger to others, self-inflicted harm, and suicide.	Assessing lethality in a distance setting, including engaging in safety planning and duty to warn in TMH settings (see Chapter 7).
3.G.14. Procedures for assessing clients' experience of trauma.	Risks in identifying appropriate assessment measures for TMH use; risk of re-traumatization with client in remote location; benefit of client being in potentially comfortable, safe, and familiar surroundings to discuss prior trauma.
3.G.15. Procedures for identifying and reporting signs of abuse and neglect.	Challenges of limited observation and non-verbal cues (e.g., odor, hygiene); challenge of confidentiality and privacy from caregiver for honest assessment in TMH settings.
3.G.16. Procedures to identify client characteristics, protective factors, risk factors, and warning signs of mental health and behavioral disorders.	Obstacles to assessing and determining a mental health diagnosis via TMH addressed (see Chapter 13).
3.G.17. Procedures for using assessment results for referral and consultation.	Confidentiality, security, and encryption of shared information, assessment results, and consultation meetings via TMH. Benefits of including multiple parties for collateral consultation via TMH (see Chapter 3).

Selecting Online Assessments

Online assessment practices should utilize assessment instruments that have been standardized and validated for online delivery. Yet many commonly used assessment measures were not normed and validated for online administration. Assessment authors and publishers are creating guidelines on the validation of or adaptation to online delivery (Corey & Ben-Porath, 2020; Krach et al., 2020; Pearson, 2021). These publications reflect ethical principles needed to administer assessments online and may even provide an evidence base for effectively using these instruments with distance delivery. Krach et al. (2020) recommend classifying assessment search results into four categories, e.g., "1) Do not use, 2) No concerns or restrictions, 3) Use with caution, and 4) No information given" (p. 929). Using this framework, CITs can approach the validation of online instruments from two angles: 1) Is/was the instrument validated for online administration, and/or 2) Is there an evidence-based literature resource that can guide ethical administration if it has not been validated for online? If the answer to both questions is "no," CITs should consider an alternative assessment measure or delivery modality.

Administering Online Assessments

Supervised versus unsupervised administration. The ACA Code of Ethics, Standard E.7.d, states, "Unless the assessment instrument is designed, intended, and validated for self-administration and/or scoring, counselors do not permit unsupervised use" (ACA, 2014, p. 12). Another term for "supervised administration" is *proctored administration*, meaning that a proctor will oversee or supervise the administration of an instrument. CITs must identify if the assessment requires proctored administration, and if so, adapt that proctored administration to online delivery with a valid evidence base that online administration will maintain the instrument's integrity.

Corey and Ben-Porath (2020) provide a "Checklist for Conducting Remote Psychological Testing Proctored via Teleconference" (p. 202). This checklist includes four "pause points:" 1) before, 2) at the start of, 3) during, and 4) after the remote testing session. Some strategies from before the session include testing equipment and software and informing the test-taker of risks and benefits. At the start of the session, they recommend confirming identity, articulating a backup plan, and verifying privacy. During the session, proctors respond to questions and maintain test security. After the session, proctors determine if the test environment was maintained and document this in test environment notes. These are only a sample of the 20-plus steps outlined by the authors, demonstrating the value of a structured guide to ensure impartial administration and to maintain the test environment's integrity.

Test environment. Administrators have a role and responsibility in monitoring the test environment. The test environment may include assessments delivered via a software system in the presence of a proctor or counselor, either in a live, in-person setting (e.g., client and counselor in the office, on a computer with pre-loaded assessment software) or virtually (via TMH). In the former setting, the proctor can maintain the test environment, minimize distractions, and maximize security in person. In the latter setting, the proctor can set expectations but may have little control over the test-taker's environment. Proctored assessments require that the proctor utilize secure software that will allow them to be virtually "present" throughout the assessment. Counselors administering online assessments where they cannot be physically present in the testing environment have a responsibility to communicate test environment expectations to the client and, if needed, family members. These include expectations of confidentiality, privacy, secure internet connections, ID checks, and other security features. The counselor conducts a test run of any technology, and clients are informed that they will be expected to scan the room to ensure it is appropriate.

Interpreting Results Online

Interpretation of test results can influence diagnoses, treatment plans, and clinical interventions. If tests are normed to be administered via technology, then CITs can utilize the procedures outlined in the administration manual. When assessments are not normed to be administered online, CITs should use caution in interpreting the results, considering their assessment of the test environment and integrity. Wright et al. (2020) remind us that no single test score should determine a clinical decision, specifying that nonstandard assessment administration, such as via TMH, broadens the margin of error. They recommend widening confidence intervals of findings and viewing results within the larger client context.

Teaching Techniques

The strategies below aim to support instruction of TMH assessment, using andragogical principles, including self-motivated learning, using prior experiences, recognizing a need for information, and immediately applying learning in a real-world context (Knowles, 1975).

1. *Reviewing Counseling Assessment Ethics.* CITs should begin with a review/refresher of counseling ethical codes that pertain to assessment and TMH. These include the ACA Code of Ethics, Standards E and H (ACA, 2014), as well as the codes of their specialization, such as ASCA, AMHCA, NCDA, NAADAC, and others.
2. *Examining Assessment Ethics Beyond Counseling.* Other professions like Psychology and Education may be more deeply rooted in assessment. Instructors and CITs can consult the *Standards for Educational and Psychological Testing* published by the American

Educational Research Association (AERA, 2014) and examine how those standards support or conflict with counseling codes.

3. *Test Development for Online Administration.* Instructors can assign CITs to research common assessments and their psychometric properties for online administration within the respective specializations. Following the framework of Corey and Ben-Porath (2020), CITs can explore whether assessment development included norms for online administration and/or if there is evidence of successful use of the instrument administered via TMH.
4. *Preparing for Proctored Online Assessment Administration.* CITs can brainstorm the steps necessary to prepare proctors to deliver assessments online. Strategies should include the actions, communication, and expectations that need to be established with the test-taker before test administration to have the most productive testing session possible.
5. *Preparing for Online Interviews and Observations.* Assessment occurs through both formal and informal measures. Informal measures may include observation and interviews. CIT can discuss and document the potential pitfalls of conducting observations and interviews online and strategies to avoid those challenges before they occur.
6. *The Impact of Errors in Online Administration.* Test administrators are required to document any variations or anomalies that occurred during the test administration in their report. CITs brainstorm the administration errors that could occur during online assessment and discuss how these errors impact the interpretation of the test results.
7. *Documenting Errors in Administration.* As established in item 6, test administrators are required to document in their report any variations or anomalies that occurred during the test administration. CITs can practice documenting the types of errors described in item 6 in formal documentation.
8. *Role-Playing Interview and Observational Assessments.* CITs can role-play (using TMH technology from Chapter 2) conducting an online assessment interview including observational components and discussing the strengths and challenges of the approach when done.
9. *Role-Playing Proctored Online Assessment.* CITs can role-play (using TMH technology from Chapter 2) conducting an online proctored

standardized assessment and discussing the strengths and challenges of the approach when done.

10. *Role-Playing Self-Administered Online Assessment.* CITs can role-play (using TMH technology from Chapter 2) conducting an online self-administered assessment with a client and discussing the strengths and challenges of the approach when done. Explore how administration may vary with a proctor-led versus self-administered online assessment.

Sample Lesson: Examining Psychometric Properties of Online Administration

Heather C. Robertson, PhD, LMHC, CRC, NCC, BC-TMH
St. John's University

Lesson Objectives

At the end of this lesson, students will have

1) examined administration manuals and published test reviews of common counseling assessments,
2) searched the literature to determine evidence to support the online administration of the assessment, and
3) analyzed their findings to determine ethical online use of selected assessments.

2024 CACREP Standards

Standards 3.G.4 (Reliability and validity in the use of assessments), 3.G.6 (Ethical and legal considerations for selecting, administering, and interpreting assessments), and 3.G.8 (Use of assessments in academic, educational, career, personal, and social development).

Materials and/or Technology Required

Students will need access to the internet and a digital database of academic content, such as those provided via university library systems.

Preparation Required

Prior instruction on identifying the reliability and validity of assessment instruments. Prior instruction on ethics of administering assessments in-person and online.

Estimated Time Required for Lesson Delivery

Prior instruction time may vary. This activity may be utilized as an out-of-class assignment or in-class activity. It is estimated that students will take 1–2 hours, depending on the depth of the literature review.

Structure and Audience for Lesson

This activity is best used in master's level counselor training in assessment. Format can be in-person or online (synchronous or asynchronous).

Lesson Content and Instructional Strategies

1. Students will be asked to identify a common assessment measure used regularly within their specialization. For example, mental health counseling students might select the Minnesota Multiphasic Personality Inventory (MMPI), whereas career counseling students might select the Strong Interest Inventory. Students may choose an instrument, or the instructor may assign it. Students may be assigned to work individually, in pairs, or in small groups.
2. Students begin by reviewing information from the publisher on the assessment. This may include the administration manual, the publisher's website, or published articles by the assessment authors on the development and validation of the assessment, including normed populations, reliability, and validity. Students should specifically seek any information on using the assessment online or through TMH modalities. Students should not confuse online assessment scoring software with administration via TMH or computerized assessment with administration via TMH. Information on the reliability and validity of the assessment via online or TMH delivery should be recorded.
3. Students will then examine any published reviews of the assessment. This may include the *Mental Measurements Yearbook* (MMY; Carlson et al., 2021), *Tests in Print* (Anderson et al., 2022), or other published reviews, e.g., National Career Development Association's *Comprehensive Guide to Career Assessments*,

Association for Assessment and Research in Counseling's *Assessment Database*. Students should specifically seek information on whether the assessment is used via online or TMH modalities. Information on the reliability and validity of the assessment via online or TMH delivery should be recorded.

4. Finally, students will conduct a peer-reviewed literature search of recent research using the instrument, specifically, the assessment via online or TMH modalities. Students should document how the instrument was adapted for online delivery and any mention of the adjustments made for delivering the assessment via TMH.
5. Using the information gathered from their research, students can assess the following: 1) Is/was the instrument validated for online administration, and/or 2) Is there an evidence-based literature resource that can guide ethical administration if it has not been validated for online? Students can utilize Krach et al. (2020) classification recommendations to determine if they would use the instrument via TMH (e.g., "1. Do not use, 2. No concerns or restrictions, 3. Use with caution, and 4. No information given," p. 929). Based on the data they found, students should be prepared to support their position.
6. The instructor can lead students in an informal sharing session or direct students to summarize their findings in a written format.

Assessment of Objectives

Assessment of the lesson objectives can be conducted formally or informally. Formally, instructors can adapt the assignment to a written paper, where students summarize their findings from items 2–5 above, including their sources and citations. Informal assessment would involve group discussion via in-person or synchronous classes or online discussion boards for asynchronous classes.

References

Anderson, N. A., Schlueter, J. E., Carlson, J. F., & Geisinger, K. F. (2022). (Eds.). *Tests in print.* Buros Center for Testing.

Carlson, J. F., & Jonson, J. L. (2021). (Eds.). *The twenty-first mental measurements yearbook.* Buros Center for Testing.

Krach, S. K., Paskiewicz, T. L., & Monk, M. M. (2020). Testing our children when the world shuts down: Analyzing recommendations for adapted tele-assessment during COVID-19. *Journal of Psychoeducational Assessment, 38*(8), 923–941. https://doi.org/10.1177/0734282920962839

Sample Lesson: Delivering Assessments via TMH: Case Study, Questions, and Discussion

Heather C. Robertson, PhD, LMHC, CRC, NCC, BC-TMH
St. John's University

Lesson Objective(s)

At the end of this lesson, students will have

1) examined a case regarding the use of delivering assessments via TMH modalities,
2) applied concepts learned in the program to the case, and
3) decided on an ethical course of action regarding the case.

2024 CACREP Standards

Standards 3.G.9 (Use of environmental assessments and systematic behavioral observations), 3.G.10 (Use of structured interviewing, symptom checklists, and personality and psychological testing), 3.G.12 (Procedures to identify substance use, addictions, and co-occurring conditions), and 3.G.13 (Procedures for assessing and responding to risk of aggression or danger to others, self-inflicted harm, and suicide).

Materials and/or Technology Required

Access to case study.

Preparation Required

Prior instruction on ethics of assessment, in person and online.

Estimated Time Required for Lesson Delivery

Prior instruction time may vary. This activity should last approximately 30–45 minutes, depending on instructional time.

Structure and Audience for Lesson

This activity is best used in master's level counselor training in assessment. Format can be in-person or online (synchronous or asynchronous).

Lesson Content and Instructional Strategies

Case Example

Taylor is a licensed professional counselor with a specialized credential in addictions counseling. They work at an outpatient substance use counseling clinic where they serve clients with both substance use and mental health concerns. Taylor provides both in-person and TMH counseling. The agency follows proper protocols for TMH, including security, encryption, state regulations, and a TMH informed consent form that complies with the ACA Code of Ethics.

Taylor has been assigned a new TMH client for intake, Client A, who presents with personal, family, and legal issues regarding cocaine use. Intake typically involves conducting a structured intake interview (Addiction Severity Index [ASI]; McLellan et al., 1992) and an assessment of motivation for treatment (University of Rhode Island Change Assessment [URICA]; McConnaughy et al., 1983). Part of the ASI requires the interviewer to assess their confidence that the respondent understands the questions and that the client is not misrepresenting their responses. The interviewer is also asked to determine whether the respondent was depressed, hostile, anxious, having trouble with reality, having difficulty with comprehension, or having suicidal thoughts during the interview. Taylor is unsure if these instruments were developed for online administration, but their supervisor instructed them to use them for the intake. They are the same instruments used during in-person intakes. Taylor read Client A's file and phone screening prior to conducting the intake but did not have any contact with Client A before the session.

Client A signed on to the intake on time but initially did not turn on the camera. Taylor asked Client A to turn on the camera, revealing that Client A was in a room that appeared to be a kitchen. Taylor asked Client A if they were in a confidential space, which they confirmed. Taylor began explaining the assessment process and what they would be doing over the next 90 minutes. Client A appeared distracted, regularly looking off-screen or at their phone. Taylor began the assessment by starting with the ASI. Client A became distressed, discouraged, and despondent when talking about their legal issues and stated they would "rather die than go back to jail." Based on these statements, Taylor decided to pause the ASI administration and conduct a Beck Depression Inventory (BDI-II; Beck et al., 1996) and a Columbia Suicide Severity Rating Scale (Posner et al., 2011) just to make sure that the client was safe and the information from the intake was accurate.

Questions

1. Assuming good intentions, what did Taylor do well? Consider their actions both before and during the assessment.
2. What ethical issues were you aware of when reading the case? Consider both those that were adhered to and those that were possible risks.
3. What thoughts, concerns, or questions do you have when you consider Taylor's preparation for the intake and the client's presentation at the start of the session?
4. What thoughts, concerns, or questions do you have when you consider Taylor's decision to stop administering the ASI and to administer the BDI-II and the CSSR?
5. What other thoughts, questions, concerns, or suggestions do you have regarding this case?

Discussion

1. Students review the case at the beginning of the lesson. The instructor may allow time for students to research the instruments in the case or provide sample copies of the instruments

(or substitute instruments) for the students to review along with the case.

2. Students can discuss the review questions above as a class, in pairs or small groups, and share their responses with the class. Online asynchronous classes may wish to use discussion boards to share their thoughts on the case.
3. The instructor can summarize the class's primary beliefs and place them into three categories: 1) did well, 2) did not do well, and 3) suggestions. This model allows students to recognize that counselors rarely act with malice, often do many things well, even if they make mistakes, and offer alternative suggestions that Taylor could have used.

Assessment of Objectives

Assessment of the lesson objectives can be conducted formally or informally. Formally, instructors can adapt the assignment to a written paper, where students review the case, research the assessments, and provide a written summary of areas in which Taylor 1) Did Well, 2) Did Not Do Well, and 3) Suggestions. Informal assessment would involve group discussion via in-person or synchronous classes or online discussion boards for asynchronous classes.

References

Beck, A. T., Steer, R. A., & Brown, G. (1996). *Beck Depression Inventory-II (BDI-II)*. APA PsycTests. https://doi.org/10.1037/t00742-000

McConnaughy, E. A., Prochaska, J. O., Velicer, W. F. (1983). Stages of change in psychotherapy: Measurement and sample profiles. *Psychotherapy: Theory, Research and Practice, 20*(3) 368–375. https://doi.org/10.1037/h0090198

McLellan A. T., Kushner H., Metzger, D., Peters, R., Smith, I., Grissom, G., Pettinati, H., & Argeriou, M. (1992). The Fifth Edition of the Addiction Severity Index. *J Subst Abuse Treat,* 9(3):199–213. https://doi.org/10.1016/0740-5472(92)90062-s

Posner, K., Brown, G. K., Stanley, B., Brent, D. A., Yershova, K. V., Oquendo, M. A., Currier, G. W., Melvin, G. A., Greenhill, L., Shen, S., & Mann, J. J. The Columbia-Suicide Severity Rating Scale: Initial validity and internal consistency findings from three multisite studies with adolescents and adults. *Am J Psychiatry, 168*(12):1266–77. https://doi.org/10.1176/appi.ajp.2011.10111704

10

Research and Program Evaluation

A counselor's engagement in research and program evaluation fluctuates depending on their role. Ethical counselors utilize evidence-based approaches in their counseling practice. Mental health counselors, school counselors, and other specialists review research for evidence-based approaches and clinical interventions. Counselor educators may engage in research as part of their role. Counselors who work with government agencies or think tanks may also engage in research, contributing knowledge to the field and advising on policy. Counselors who work as program directors, division leaders, or external auditors regularly engage in program evaluation.

When research and program evaluation services are conducted online or via distance technologies, counselors adapt their research activities to telemental health (TMH) parameters. Based on these varied situations, counselors-in-training (CITs) need to understand the unique elements of research when engaging in distance practices.

Key Concepts

CACREP Standards

CACREP Section 3.H, Research and Program Evaluation, outlines 11 learning outcomes in relation to research and program evaluation (CACREP, 2024, p. 16). Much like the standard on assessment, none of the changes or updates specifically address the use of TMH or distance research. The 2024 version expands its definition of research beyond quantitative, qualitative, and mixed-methods to include practice-based and action research. The inclusion of practice-based research suggests that as practices expand to TMH, practice-based research will also extend to TMH settings. Action-based research supports Knowles's principles of andragogy, involving applying learning in real-world contexts (1975). Table 10.1 provides examples of how TMH can be infused into research and program evaluation standards. If suggested concepts are unfamiliar, the instructor is encouraged to explore the training and reading materials suggested in Chapter 1.

Table 10.1

CACREP Section 3.H (Research and Program Evaluation) and Suggested TMH Content

CACREP Standards (2024)	Suggested TMH Content
3.H.1. The importance of research in advancing the counseling profession, including the use of research to inform counseling practice.	Benefit of online research in reaching a wider range of respondents in varied and remote locations; ability to survey people beyond our immediate region/reach (Hooley & Dodd, 2016).
3.H.2. Identification and evaluation of the evidence base for counseling theories, interventions, and practices.	While examining evidence-base for theories and interventions, explore evidence for using theories in TMH contexts.
3.H.3. Qualitative, quantitative, and mixed methods research designs.	Exploration of various types of technology for conducting research, such as online instruments (see Chapter 9), recorded interviews, and automatic transcription services.

CACREP Standards (2024)	Suggested TMH Content
3.H.4. Practice-based and action research methods.	Capacity for TMH to record interactions between clients/counselors (e.g., audio, video, transcript, text, email) to support practice-based and action research (with permissions).
3.H.5. Statistical tests used in conducting research and program evaluation.	Issues of access, ease, and accuracy of conducting analyses via statistical software for both in-person and online research.
3.H.6. Analysis and use of data in research.	Technology utilized to support quantitative and qualitative analysis (e.g., SPSS, NVivo) during research, and the importance of security of 3rd-party software (e.g., encryption, storage, Business Associate Agreements) for both in-person and online research.
3.H.7. Use of research methods and procedures to evaluate counseling interventions.	Benefit of TMH observations, transcripts, and recording in research as opposed to client/counselor recall.
3.H.8. Program evaluation designs and procedures, including needs assessments, formative assessments, and summative assessments to inform decision-making and advocacy.	Examining the appropriate administration of needs assessments, formative assessments, and summative assessments via online methods (see Chapter 9), as well as security of retrieving program data from online databases.
3.H.9. Culturally sustaining and developmentally relevant outcome measures for counseling services.	Capacity for TMH research to capture perspectives and experiences of diverse audiences (see Chapter 4).
3.H.10. Ethical and legal considerations relevant to conducting, interpreting, and reporting the results of research and program evaluation.	Adherence to ethical standards for both research guidelines and TMH guidelines; focus on the safety, security, and storage of research data.
3.H.11. Culturally sustaining and developmentally responsive strategies for conducting, interpreting, and reporting the results of research and program evaluation.	Recognizing limitations of online services based on digital access, cultural divides, or developmental ability (see Chapter 4). Propensity for TMH research to exclude populations without access to technology.

Using Online Research Tools Safely

Online researchers must utilize precautions to minimize risk. One of the primary concerns among research respondents is the confidentiality and anonymity of their responses. While online survey tools and standardized measures appear anonymous, many automatically collect **internet protocol (IP) addresses**, which can be traced back to an individual server and their identity. Many tools can turn off the IP address collection to maintain the anonymity of the respondents. Using third-party tools raises the question of who owns the data collected via these tools and who is responsible for a data breach. Researchers must also examine the security of online data storage, such as cloud storage systems. These issues are addressed in the informed consent document so that respondents are made fully aware of the risks of engaging in online research.

Online library databases are one example of accessing online information to facilitate research, such as meta-analyses. Government agencies, such as the U.S. Bureau of Labor Statistics (BLS), have large data sets that are accessible to the public. The ability to access data from online sources requires researcher discernment, ethics, and judgment. It is the researcher's responsibility to vet the validity of these sources and the data provided. Researchers reference the timeliness of the data, as older data may not accurately represent the current situation. Using current data to represent older trends would be a misrepresentation. Researchers note conflicts of interest among the entities posting the data and their vested interest in presenting it through a particular lens (e.g., tobacco or pharmaceutical companies minimizing the risks of their products). Search engines use artificial intelligence (AI) to generate data responses, and the researcher is responsible for analyzing the source of the information for accuracy and authenticity.

Social Media and Open Forums in Online Research

Expanding amounts of information are posted online via social media sites, blogs, and other online forums. According to a Pew Research study, 81% of internet user respondents use YouTube, 69% use Facebook, 40% use Instagram, and another 25% use X (formerly Twitter), WhatsApp, and TikTok (Auxier & Anderson, 2021). Social media research may include a) collecting responses via social media platforms, b) utilizing data posted on social media for research, c) publishing research findings on social media, or d) utilizing research findings reported on social media. Phillips (2011) states that social media research could help many psychology researchers reach beyond the common pool of undergraduate students while citing some common pitfalls of social media research. One of these pitfalls is using one's personal social media account to gather findings instead of creating separate accounts for social media research. In addition, Phillips (2011) cites the struggle of collecting demographic information when conducting social media research.

Regarding the use of posted and published research on social media, Zimba and Gasparyan (2021) specify that professionals in the field should moderate sites and that authors may promote their publications via social media to gain more visibility in the field. Most universities have recognized social media research's potential and have created protocols or policies within their Institutional Review Boards (IRBs) specific to social media research (see samples in reference list, e.g., Penn State University, University of Maine). A prudent first step for any online researcher would be to check their university and IRB policies surrounding social media research.

Teaching Techniques

The strategies below support TMH research and program evaluation instruction, using andragogical principles, including self-motivated learning, using prior experiences, recognizing a need for information, and immediately applying learning in a real-world context (Knowles, 1975).

1. *Reviewing Counseling Research Ethics.* CITs should begin with a review/refresher of counseling ethical codes that pertain to research and TMH. These include the ACA Code of Ethics (2014), Standards G and H, as well as codes of their specialization, such as ASCA, AMHCA, NCDA, NAADAC, and others.
2. *Exploring the Security of Online Survey Tools.* Online researchers often utilize survey tools created by third parties in their research. Instructors can assign CITs to examine posted information on the security of these tools, including data encryption, data storage, and data ownership. CITs can examine the difference in security features between paid survey tools (e.g., Qualtrics, Survey Monkey) versus free survey systems (e.g., Google Forms), as well as policies on data breaches.
3. *Transitioning Research to TMH Delivery.* CITs are often asked to design research proposals or examine a research study as a part of their training. Instructors can have CITs reconsider how a study

would be altered if administered via TMH as a component of that assignment. CITs can discuss any additional strategies needed, as well as consider data security if data were to be collected, stored, and processed online.

4. *Designing Quantitative TMH Research.* CITs can design a quantitative study to be administered via TMH. Examples include survey research or administering standardized assessments (see Chapter 9). CITs should consider quantitative TMH data collection methods, which statistical measures would be needed for analysis, any third-party software used in the study, and how the data would be collected, analyzed, and stored via technology.
5. *Designing Qualitative TMH Research.* CITs can design a qualitative study to be administered via TMH. Examples might include interviews or observations (see Chapter 9). CITs should consider qualitative TMH data collection methods, which procedures would be used for analysis, any third-party software used in the study, and how the data would be collected, analyzed, and stored via technology.
6. *Practice-Based and Action TMH Research.* Discuss and explore the ethical use of practice-based and action research with counseling clients. Some questions to explore include: What considerations should be made when engaging our clients and students in action-based research? How might those considerations vary when we use TMH practice-based research (e.g., researching clients and students engaged in TMH services)? How might the use of recorded sessions vary from data collected via surveys, assessments, observations, or interviews? How might data collection and storage change?
7. *Social Media Research.* Discuss and explore the ethical use of social media research; consider both collecting information already posted and recruiting social media respondents. Some questions to explore include: What considerations should be made when engaging in social media research? What additional cautions might need to be considered when collecting data from social media posts or recruiting social media respondents? What policies exist at your institution on social media research, if any?
8. *Examining Online Databases.* Counseling researchers examine all types of issues. CITs can select issues they might want to research and brainstorm online data resources to support their research. These might include literature or other information databases,

such as those posted by government agencies. Instructors can ask CITs to examine these online databases and conduct an assessment of their validity, authenticity, and conflicting interests.

9. *Online Program Evaluation.* Depending on their specialization (e.g., school, community mental health centers), CITs can discuss what data would be needed to help them evaluate the effectiveness of the counseling services provided. CITs can consider where or how they might obtain the necessary data for their program evaluation, including examining existing records, surveying respondents, or other means. Once CITs have developed a plan for program evaluation, instructors can have them adapt that plan to TMH program evaluation, where CITs collect and analyze data in an online setting. Discuss and explore how their program evaluation plan would vary if they could only use TMH program evaluation methods.
10. *Examining the Accuracy of Online Transcription Services.* Many qualitative researchers use online transcription services when documenting interviews to transcribe interview data. Many technological tools discussed in Chapter 2 also provide transcription services and recording. Instructors can have students use online recording and transcription services to assess the accuracy of the information. Because qualitative research often involves member checking as a validity measure, CITs can practice member checking by auditing transcripts for the accuracy of the information, as they would need to do when conducting online research.

Sample Lesson: Integrating AI in Counseling Research: Utilizing ChatGPT for Literature Review and Research Question Development

Nouna Jalilzadeh, PhD, LMHC, NCC
St. John's University

Lesson Objectives

The purpose of this lesson is to encourage students to embrace technology, ethically and responsibly, in the counseling research process. At the end of this lesson, students will have

1) examined the ACA Code of Ethics,
2) demonstrated and identified ethical considerations and implications of utilizing artificial intelligence (AI) in counseling research,
3) developed proficiency in using ChatGPT or other AI technology for literature review assistance, and
4) formulate research questions.

2024 CACREP Standards

Standards 3.H.1 (Advancing the counseling profession, including the use of research to inform counseling practice) and 3.H.10 (Ethical and legal considerations relevant to conducting, interpreting, and reporting the results of research and program evaluation).

Materials and/or Technology Required

ChatGPT or other AI technology. If the lesson is being delivered in person, students will need to bring laptops or other devices to access ChatGPT/AI. At least half of the students should have an account with ChatGPT/AI technology. Access to samples of research proposals, databases for literature review, and the ACA Code of Ethics is needed.

Preparation Required

Students should have a foundational knowledge of conducting research, research methodologies, ethical considerations in research, and a basic understanding of ChatGPT or AI technology. Prior exposure to literature review writing is recommended.

Estimated Time Required for Lesson Delivery

Approximately 60–90 minutes. If delivered online synchronously or asynchronously, students can work independently or in pairs; however, if working independently, each must have access to ChatGPT/AI technology.

Structure and Audience for Lesson

This activity is best used in in-person or online synchronous classroom settings, including master's, doctoral, or professional development training. However, adaptations can be made for online asynchronous learning via a learning management system (LMS) and recorded videos, discussion boards, and video presentations.

Lesson Content and Instructional Strategies

1. The instructor provides instructional content to students with an overview of research in counseling, ethical considerations guiding research practices, and ethics pertaining to the incorporation of AI into counseling research.
2. The instructor introduces the role of AI, specifically ChatGPT, and discusses potential benefits, challenges, and ethical considerations of using ChatGPT/AI for research purposes, literature review assistance, and development of research questions.
3. The instructor introduces the activity as a way for students to utilize technology ethically, responsibly, and critically to assist with literature review and research question development.
4. Depending on the number of students, students can work individually, in pairs, or in groups where at least one member can access ChatGPT/AI software.
5. For this activity, students are asked to use ChatGPT/AI software to 1) write a literature review outline for a specific counseling topic and 2) develop research question/s based on the written literature review outline.
6. Individuals, pairs, or groups are asked to choose a research topic (e.g., cultural considerations when counseling undocumented immigrants) and initiate a literature review outline utilizing ChatGPT/AI.
7. Students provide an initial prompt to the ChatGPT/AI software, such as "generate a literature review outline on cultural considerations when counseling undocumented immigrants."
8. After receiving their initial response, students use the ACA Code of Ethics, including content on Research Responsibilities, review at least three peer-reviewed journals on the topic, and have ChatGPT edit the document and enhance the output as necessary and relevant to their specific topic. For example, "edit to include information on undocumented immigrants with Middle Eastern backgrounds."
9. Based on what the software generates, students add elements to their literature review outline until they feel they have a comprehensive outline that they are satisfied with.
10. After completing the literature review outline, students are asked to formulate research question/s for their counseling research utilizing ChatGPT/AI.

11. Students provide a prompt to the ChatGPT/AI software, such as "generate a research question on cultural considerations when counseling undocumented immigrants."
12. Based on what the software formulates, students refine their research questions using ethical guidelines, ask follow-up questions, and edit their specific research focus until they feel confident in their research question.
13. After enough time, the instructor brings the group back together for a final discussion/reflection.
14. Each individual, pair, or group will present their literature review outline and research questions and answer the following questions:
    a. What were your most significant challenges while using ChatGPT for literature review assistance and research question formulation?
    b. While refining your literature review or research question, how did you navigate ethical considerations specific to counseling research?
    c. Were there any unexpected insights or valuable contributions from ChatGPT that positively influenced your literature review or research question?
    d. Reflecting on the overall experience, do you believe that AI tools like ChatGPT can enhance the efficiency and creativity of the counseling research process? Why or why not?
    e. Were there instances where you felt the need to override or modify the suggestions provided by ChatGPT due to ethical concerns or considerations specific to counseling? Can you provide examples?
    f. Thinking about future applications, how might you use the insights gained from this activity in your counseling research endeavors or professional practice?
    g. What suggestions do you have for improving or refining the activity to better align with the ethical considerations and challenges in counseling research?
    h. Other comments about the experience.

Assessment of Objectives

Lesson objectives will be assessed via the classroom discussion and the students' responses to the activity. Instructors may also require students to submit their activity (e.g., download a transcript from AI with multiple variations) as evidence of their engagement. Pairs and groups can also perform peer review, look at one another's literature review outline and research questions, and provide feedback.

Sample Lesson: Online Quantitative and Qualitative Research in Counseling

Gina Cicco, EdD, LMHC, NCC, Certified School Counselor
St. John's University

Lesson Objectives

At the end of this lesson, students will be able to

1) identify the key features of quantitative and qualitative research methods,
2) distinguish between quantitative and qualitative research designs,
3) provide examples of the different types of quantitative and qualitative research methodologies, and
4) discuss ethical use of technology in online counseling research studies.

2024 CACREP Standards

Standard 3.H.3 (Qualitative, quantitative, and mixed methods research designs).

Materials and/or Technology Required

A videoconference platform such as Zoom, Teams, or WebEx; PowerPoint; learning management system such as Canvas or Blackboard.

Preparation Required

Students will be assigned to read the ACA Code of Ethics (Section G, Research and Publication) and chapters 10, 11, 14, and 15 in Erford

(2024). The reading assignments and corresponding review questions will be posted on the LMS at the course's start or two weeks before the synchronous lesson.

Estimated Time Required for Lesson Delivery

2–3 hours.

Structure and Audience for Lesson

Synchronous online setting, graduate students.

Lesson Content and Instructional Strategies

Delivery of PowerPoint presentation and short videos.

1. The instructor will discuss the hallmarks of both quantitative and qualitative research paradigms and provide critical comparisons and contrasts between the two, including objectivity versus subjectivity, generalizability, question formulation, researcher role, cause/effect relationships, making meaning of contexts, data collection and instrumentation, and confirmatory versus exploratory studies. A PowerPoint presentation and a short online video on the topic will be employed to summarize the initial discussion.
2. Quantitative research designs and general quantitative methods will be outlined in the context of non-experimental versus experimental designs.
3. Descriptive, associational, and comparative/group difference quantitative designs will be explained, and a brief introduction to descriptive and inferential statistics will be provided.
4. Four major qualitative research designs and methods will be outlined: ethnography, phenomenology, grounded theory, and case studies.
5. The instructor will summarize the major tenets of the two major research paradigms by creating a live chart to be filled in and completed with the help of students responding to comprehension questions. The chart will be displayed as a working document in the synchronous presentation and serve as a review/study sheet and assessment method.
6. Once the chart is complete, the instructor will lead a discussion on the impact of online research on the methods discussed.

Students will be asked to explore how using these various methodologies in online research settings may impact research design, as well as data storage, analysis, and interpretation of results. These elements can be added to the chart called "online research considerations."

Assessment of Objectives

1. Students will be questioned for comprehension of objectives throughout the lesson.
2. Students' responses during the chart formulation will also indicate their comprehension of the lecture and discussion sections of the lesson.
3. Students will be sent into three breakout rooms to work on a small-group assignment, and the group reporter will later present the work of their respective groups to the larger group as a whole. Each group will designate a recorder and reporter. Creativity in presentations will be encouraged.

    a. Group 1 will list key quantitative and qualitative research paradigm features, highlighting researcher roles.
    b. Group 2 will provide the major distinctions between quantitative and qualitative research designs.
    c. Group 3 will list and briefly explain examples of quantitative and qualitative research designs.
    d. All groups will discuss, brainstorm, document, and share the benefits and challenges of conducting quantitative and qualitative research via technology in relation to content from the lecture, the Erford text, and the ACA Code of Ethics. These findings should be addressed in their PowerPoint presentations.

References

American Counseling Association. (2014). *Code of ethics.* American Counseling Association. https://www.counseling.org/knowledge-center/ethics

Erford, B. T. (2024). *Research and evaluation in counseling* (3rd ed.). Cognella.

Entry-Level
Specialized Practice Area

11

Addictions Counseling

Addictions counseling is currently recognized as a specialization within the counseling profession. Still, there is ongoing discussion about whether tr aining in addictions counseling should be separate from other counseling specializations or embedded into all counseling (Morgen et al., 2012). The importance of substance use counseling is embedded throughout the CACREP Foundational Counseling Curriculum, as evidenced by Standards 3.C.5 (Lifespan Development, theories and neurobiological etiology of addictions), and 3.G.12 (Assessment and diagnosis, procedures to identify substance use, addictions, and co-occurring conditions; CACREP, 2024). In addition, CACREP recognizes the role of addictions counseling as a stand-alone profession, distinct from other specializations with which it regularly overlaps, such as clinical mental health counseling or clinical rehabilitation counseling.

Addictions counseling encompasses more than substance use disorders (SUD), including process addictions, such as gambling, eating, shopping, internet use, and other problematic behaviors. While the *DSM-5-TR* only lists "Gambling Disorder" (F63.0) as a non-substance-related disorder, other addictive behavior could be considered "Other Specified Disruptive, Impulse Control, and Conduct Disorders" (F91.8), depending on the impact it has on the person's functioning and overall wellbeing (American Psychiatric Association, 2022). Like other counseling specializations, addictions counseling occurs in both face-to-face (F2F) and telemental health contexts (TMH). As such, addictions counselors-in-training (CITs) need to learn how to practice in a TMH setting.

Key Concepts

CACREP Standards

CACREP Section 5.A (Entry-Level Specialized Practice Areas, Addiction Counseling) outlines 13 learning outcomes concerning addictions counseling. Like other sections of the standards, this specialization does not specifically address the use of TMH delivery. However, there are distinct and discernable connections to content on TMH in the addictions counseling curriculum, as outlined in Table 11.1. If these concepts are unfamiliar, the instructor is encouraged to explore the training and reading materials suggested in Chapter 1.

Table 11.1

CACREP Section 5.A (Addictions Counseling) and Suggested TMH Content

CACREP Standards (2024)	Suggested TMH Content
5.A.1. Neurological, behavioral, psychological, physical, and social effects of psychoactive substances and addictive disorders on the user and significant others.	Capacity for non-substance behaviors (e.g., shopping, gambling, internet use—all facilitated by technology) to trigger pleasure hormones (e.g., dopamine, serotonin) like substance use (Smith, 2015).
5.A.2. Risk and protective factors for substance use disorders.	Risk of technology perpetuating addictive behaviors (e.g., gambling, shopping, pornography viewing) while simultaneously providing access to online support/therapy as a protective factor.
5.A.3. Assessment for symptoms of psychoactive substance toxicity, intoxication, and withdrawal.	Challenges in assessing substance use and active use when using TMH due to limitation of counselor's senses (e.g., sight, smell).
5.A.4. Strategies for enhancing client motivation to change, managing cravings, and preventing relapse.	Wearable technology, online, and self-management tools can be used to support recovery and connect clients to treatment.

CACREP Standards (2024)	Suggested TMH Content
5.A.5. Abstinence and harm reduction models of addiction recovery.	Benefits/challenges of TMH in toxicology and accessing harm reduction (see below).
5.A.6. Evaluating and identifying individualized strategies and treatment modalities relative to substance use disorder severity, stages of change, or recovery.	TMH addictions groups can connect clients at various stages of recovery, support of effective treatment group sizes (e.g., too large or too small). Assessing if TMH treatment is appropriate depending on stage of recovery.
5.A.7. Pharmacological interventions used to address substance use withdrawal, craving, and relapse prevention.	Understanding medication-assisted treatment (MAT) and the benefits of and/or risks in providing MAT via TMH (e.g., methadone monitoring; Weintraub et al., 2018).
5.A.8. Substance use recovery service delivery modalities and networks within the continuum of care, such as primary care, outpatient, partial treatment, inpatient, integrated behavioral healthcare, and aftercare.	Capacity for TMH to enhance addictions treatment across service delivery modalities, e.g., outpatient treatment, collateral and family involvement for inpatient settings, and medical collaboration for integrated care (Celio et al., 2017; Molfenter et al., 2018).
5.A.9. Recovery support tools and systems to include vocation, family, social networks, and community systems in the addiction treatment and recovery process.	Capacity for TMH to enhance wraparound services for recovery treatment, including collaborating with professionals and family (Molfenter et al., 2018); TMH with families (see Chapter 16), rehabilitation counseling (see Chapter 13), and vocational counseling (see Chapters 6 and 12); 24/7 12-step support groups via TMH.
5.A.10. Culturally and developmentally relevant education programs that raise awareness and support addiction and substance use prevention and the recovery process.	Capacity for TMH addiction treatment to reach diverse clients/counselors, coupled with limits to technology access based on race, education, and income (see Chapter 4).

CACREP Standards (2024)	Suggested TMH Content
5.A.11. Regulatory processes, continuum of care, and service delivery in addiction counseling.	Attention to the Association for Addiction Professionals' standards for e-therapy; awareness of state laws and federal regulation 42 CFR-Part 2 that regulate addiction treatment via TMH.
5.A.12. Strategies for interfacing with the legal system and working with court-referred clients.	Encryption and security in transmitting and communicating court-ordered reports (e.g., probation reports) via the **Health Insurance Portability and Accountability Act** (HIPAA), **electronic protected health information (ePHI)**, and federal regulation 42 CFR-Part 2 standards.
5.A.13. Third-party reimbursement and other practice and management issues in addictions counseling.	Insurance, Medicaid, and Medicare reimbursement models for SUD and addictions; restrictions to reimbursement and/or state funding for TMH service delivery.

Efficacy, Legal, and Ethical Concerns

Addiction treatment was already effectively utilizing TMH before the pandemic (Celio et al., 2017; Huskamp et al., 2018), including treatment of gambling disorders (Carlbring et al., 2012) and co-occurring disorders (Jaconis et al., 2017). Some interventions included wearable apps for alcohol use monitoring (Barrio et al., 2017). Twelve-step groups, such as Alcoholics Anonymous (AA), Narcotics Anonymous (NA), Overeaters Anonymous (OA), and Gamblers Anonymous (GA), utilized phone meetings, video meetings, and chat-based/message board meetings before the pandemic. Virtual self-help communities offer 24-hour meetings around triggering holidays (e.g., New Year's Eve, Thanksgiving). Online resources are praised as a complement to F2F treatment and help individuals in recovery stay connected to a support group 24/7.

Addictions counseling is protected by HIPAA and federal regulation 42 CFR-Part 2. Cautions like safety, security, encryption, and emergency planning also apply to TMH addiction counseling. Addiction counselors need to be aware of federal, state, and local guidelines directing TMH treatment, as many addiction recovery centers are publicly funded and held to additional standards.

The International Association of Addictions and Offender Counselors (IAAOC) is the division of ACA focused on addictions counseling. IAAOC specifies that its members follow the ACA Code of Ethics in their practice. The Association for Addiction Professionals, also known as NAADAC, is a broader professional development organization for addictions professionals. NAADAC encompasses the National Certification Commission for Addiction Professionals (NCC AP), which grants national certifications in addictions counseling, such as the Master Addictions Counselor (MAC), National Certified Addiction Counselor (NCAC), and others. The NAADAC/NCC AP Ethical Standards were updated in 2021, including Principle VI: E-therapy, E-supervision, and Social Media, which includes 20 different standards that address TMH and addictions counseling.

TMH Addictions Counseling Benefits and Challenges

A primary benefit of TMH during the pandemic was the ability for clients to continue addiction treatment despite stay-at-home orders (Mark et al., 2021). During COVID-19, substance use facilities increased TMH treatment across the country, ranging from an 84% increase in services in the South to a 246% increase in services in the Northeast (Cantor et al., 2021). The ability to continue care supports relapse prevention and reduces return-to-use behaviors. While online 12-step groups provide support, some clients choose not to use them, and others benefit from continued 1:1 or group counseling sessions.

Assessment may be part of the addiction counselor's responsibilities. TMH services limit observational skills and olfactory senses, which may be needed for an accurate assessment or mental status exam (MSE). Telephone, email, or text sessions do not allow an addiction counselor to see the client's appearance, which can provide cues to the substance use patterns. Other precautions needed for assessment are addressed in Chapter 9.

Alcohol and drug treatment facilities that utilize abstinence models often use toxicology screenings (e.g., drug testing) conducted via urine samples, saliva swabs, breathalyzers, or other mechanisms to measure ingested substance levels. One challenge of TMH treatment in an abstinence setting is scheduling toxicology screenings when clients are not physically in the office. In harm reduction models, treatment may include medication-assisted treatment (MAT), such as prescribing suboxone or naltrexone. Methadone is distributed via structured clinics on a daily or periodic basis. Harm reduction centers distribute clean needles, fentanyl test strips, naloxone, and other recovery tools. Harm reduction providers using TMH, where clients are not physically in an office, need other means to distribute these medications or materials that are critical to client safety and recovery.

Teaching Techniques

The strategies below support instruction of TMH within addictions counseling, using andragogical principles, including self-motivated learning, using prior experiences, recognizing a need for information, and immediately applying learning in a real-world context (Knowles, 1975).

1. *Reviewing Addictions TMH Counseling Ethics.* CITs (counselors-in-training) should begin with a review/refresher of counseling ethical codes that pertain to addictions counseling and TMH. These include the ACA Code of Ethics, Section H, Distance Counseling (ACA, 2014), and the updated NAADAC/NCC AP Ethical Standards, including Principle VI: E-therapy, E-supervision, and Social Media. Instructors and CITs can explore areas in which the codes are complimentary and conflicting concerning TMH and addictions counseling.
2. *42 CFR-Part 2 and TMH Addictions Counseling.* Addictions CITs should be familiar with the federal regulations specified in 42 CFR-Part 2 pertaining to confidentiality and addictions treatment. Instructors can have CITs examine *Substance Use Confidentiality Regulations* on the Substance Abuse and Mental Health Services Administration (SAMHSA) website specific to TMH and identify how TMH is addressed or excluded in the law: https://www.samhsa.gov/about-us/who-we-are/laws-regulations/confidentiality-regulations-faqs
3. *Clients Under the Influence.* Addictions counselors need to address active substance use with their clients or confront clients who appear to be under the influence. Instructors and CITs can discuss the signs and symptoms that they might recognize in a TMH session that signal that a client is potentially under the influence of substances. Consider different TMH modalities, including phone, video, email, and text. Students can brainstorm and role play how they would address potential substance use with clients in a TMH session.
4. *Conducting Addictions Assessments.* Addictions counselors regularly assess clients' substance use, which may include evaluating current and prior use, as well as assessing safety, such as in the

role of substance abuse professionals (SAP). Consider different types of addictions assessment (e.g., standardized measures, intake interviews, observations, toxicology samples). Discuss and explore how these assessment practices might vary when conducted via TMH. What pitfalls can occur, and what additional steps/stages are needed to ensure an effective assessment?

5. *Online Self-Help Groups.* Twelve-step groups (e.g., AA, NA, GA, OA) are regularly praised for connecting clients to recovery support nearly 24/7 via multiple modalities (e.g., video, phone, chat). Because 12-step groups are led by peers instead of professional counselors, they are not classified as counseling groups but as support groups. Instructors and CITs can discuss/debate the risks and benefits of online 12-step support groups in treatment.
6. *TMH Abstinence Models.* Abstinence recovery models typically require that the client refrain from all substances or minimally refrain from using their drug of choice. One way in which abstinence-based treatment programs monitor use is via toxicology samples that require a person to appear in person. Instructors and CITs can discuss/debate the risks and benefits of using TMH in abstinence-based recovery programs and alternative methods of monitoring abstinence.
7. *TMH Harm Reduction Models.* Harm reduction recovery models advocate for reduced substance use and/or safe substance use if someone elects to use. Harm reduction programs may participate in needle exchanges or administer fentanyl test strips, as well as conducting psychoeducation and connecting individuals to community resources to support people in recovery. Instructors and CITs can discuss/debate the risks and benefits of using TMH in harm reduction recovery programs.
8. *TMH and MAT.* Medication-assisted treatment (MAT) supports people in recovery with medication to block, mimic, or reduce substance use symptoms. Some MAT protocols are closely monitored (e.g., daily methadone distribution), while others require less interaction (e.g., once-a-month injection of naltrexone). Consider MAT and TMH treatment. Instructors and CITs can explore, discuss, and debate when TMH treatment is appropriate based on the level of care (LOC) and whether MAT provides a risk or benefit to client treatment at that level.
9. *Process Addictions.* Many process addictions are facilitated by technology. Examples include excessive and "out of control"

online gambling, online shopping, online pornography viewing, and internet use. TMH uses technology to facilitate treatment. Instructors and CITs can explore, discuss, and debate the use of TMH treatment with technology-facilitated addiction. CITs can identify different cases and conditions where TMH may not be an appropriate treatment based on technology-related behavior.

10. *Legal Interactions.* Clients in addiction treatment occasionally have legal concerns related to their substance use. These legal concerns may include driving infractions, parenting and custody issues, or other felonies/misdemeanors related to substance use and criminal behavior. How can TMH be both a benefit and a risk to those with legal infractions? Consider the ways counselors might be required to interact with legal personnel. What cautions must be utilized to protect client confidentiality while providing information needed for their legal concerns when communicating via technology or providing treatment via TMH?

Sample Lesson: Online Assessment for Addiction Disorders

Leo Gonzalez, PhD, LMHC, NCC
St. John's University

Lesson Objectives

At the end of this lesson, students will have

1) explored multiple assessments for addiction,
2) evaluated these assessments for online administration, and
3) discussed the pros and cons of assessing substance use disorders online.

2024 CACREP Standards

Standards 3.G.12 (Procedures to identify substance use, addictions, and co-occurring conditions), 3.G.5 (Culturally sustaining and developmental considerations for selecting, administering, and interpreting assessments, including individual accommodations and environmental modifications), and 5.A.3 (Assessment for symptoms of psychoactive substance toxicity, intoxication, and withdrawal).

Materials or Technology Required

Internet access.

Preparation Required

1) Students should have a foundational understanding of addiction and assessment practices, as well as the impact of technology on assessment.
2) The instructor should be familiar with the websites and resources in this lesson. It is recommended that, before the lesson, the instructor review the sites and assessments that students will be exploring.

Estimated Time Required for Lesson Delivery

Approximately 60 minutes.

Structure and Audience for Lesson

This activity is designed for in-person or online instruction. The intended audience is master's students enrolled in addictions counseling programs or learning about addiction assessment.

Lesson Content and Instructional Strategies

1. Students will work individually, in pairs or small groups. At least one member of each group/pair must have a device with internet access. Breakout rooms or discussion boards can be used for online synchronous and asynchronous instruction.
2. The instructor will direct students to the National Institute on Drug Abuse (NIDA) Screening and Assessment Tools Chart, as well as SAMHSA's Appendix C–Screening and Assessments (see Additional Resources). These two resources contain links or information on ten assessments including Screening to Brief Intervention (S2BI); Brief Screening for Alcohol, Tobacco, and Other Drugs (BSTAD); Tobacco, Alcohol, Prescription Medication and other Substance Use Tool (TAPS); Alcohol Screening and Brief Intervention for Youth: A Practitioner's Guide (NIAAA); Opioid Risk Tool-OUD (ORT-OUD Chart); Alcohol Use Disorders Identification Test (AUDIT); The Short Michigan Alcoholism Screening Test (SMAST); MAST-Geriatric Version (MAST-G); The Problem Oriented Screening Instrument for Teenagers (POSIT);

The Self-Administered Alcohol Screening (SAAST); and the Addiction Research Foundation Clinical Institute Withdrawal Assessment for Alcohol (CIWA-Ar).

3. Each student/group/pair will select or be assigned one SUD assessment or screening tool to review. Each student/group/pair should select or be assigned a different assessment and screening measure to minimize duplication. Each student/group/pair will work for 20–30 minutes to thoroughly review the selected assessment and record their responses to the following questions:
   a. What is the purpose of the assessment/screening tool? Who is it designed for?
   b. What information is available on the administration of the assessment? How is it designed to be administered, e.g., for example, in person, online, by a clinician, self-report, or another way?
   c. Can you locate any information (on this page or other sources) on whether the tool is appropriate to be administered online via TMH? If yes, what information could you find?
   d. After reviewing the instrument, what concerns would you have about administering it online instead of in-person?
   e. How would the severity of the person's response impact your concerns about administering it online? In other words, would you be as comfortable using the instrument with someone who screened for low substance use as you would be with someone who screened for high substance use? Why or why not?
   f. In the context of TMH assessments for addiction disorders, how does culture influence the process? What strategies would you implement to tailor your telehealth assessment methods to accommodate the cultural nuances and ensure the efficacy of treatment for your diverse client base?
4. After 20–30 minutes, the instructor reconvenes the class for group sharing and discussion. Students will share the results of their evaluation with the group, verbally or using visual cues.
5. After all students/groups/pairs have shared, the instructor reminds students that formal assessment and screening measures are only one type of assessment. Another assessment measure is clinical interview and observation. Students are asked to consider and share how online administration may impact clinical

interviews and observations during the assessment process (e.g., odor, pupil dilation, gait, toxicology testing, communication patterns).

6. The instructor closes the lessons by asking students to brainstorm responses to the following questions. Responses can be recorded and shared as a group/class, or individually and reported out to the larger class:
   a. What are the pros and cons of administering addiction assessments online?
   b. What must you consider when engaging in online assessment for SUD?
   c. As a counselor, how can you practice ethical and effective online assessment for SUD, including both formal and informal assessments?

Assessment of Objective

The lesson objective will be assessed via classroom discussion and the students' responses to the activity. Students may also be asked to submit their responses to both small group work and larger brainstorming sessions.

References

National Institute on Drug Abuse (NIDA). (2023, January 6). Screening and assessment tools chart. https://nida.nih.gov/nidamed-medical-health-professionals/screening-tools-resources/chart-screening-tools

Substance Abuse and Mental Health Services Administration (SAMHSA). Center for Substance

Abuse Treatment. (1997). *A Guide to Substance Abuse Services for Primary Care Clinicians. Treatment Improvement Protocol (TIP) Series, No. 24. Appendix C—Screening and Assessment Instruments.* https://www.ncbi.nlm.nih.gov/books/NBK64829/

Sample Lesson: TMH Addictions Counseling: Case Study, Questions, and Discussion

Heather C. Robertson, PhD, LMHC, CRC, NCC, BC-TMH
St. John's University

Lesson Objectives

At the end of this lesson, students will have

1) examined a case on delivering TMH addictions counseling,
2) applied concepts learned in the program to the case, and
3) decided on an ethical course of action regarding the case.

2024 CACREP Standards

Standards 5.A.3 (Assessment for symptoms of psychoactive substance toxicity, intoxication, and withdrawal) and 5.A.7 (Pharmacological interventions used to address substance use withdrawal, craving, and relapse prevention).

Materials and/or Technology Required

Access to case study.

Preparation Required

Prior instruction on TMH and addictions counseling.

Estimated Time Required for Lesson Delivery

Prior instruction time may vary. Depending on instructional time, this activity should last approximately 30–45 minutes.

Structure and Audience for Lesson

This activity is best used in master's level counselor training in addictions counseling. Format can be in-person, or online (synchronous or asynchronous).

Lesson Content and Instructional Strategies

Case Example

In Chapter 9, you met Taylor, a licensed professional counselor with a specialized credential in addictions counseling. They work at an outpatient substance use counseling clinic, serving clients with substance use and mental health concerns. They provide both in-person and TMH counseling. The agency follows proper protocols for TMH, including security, encryption, state regulations, and a TMH informed consent form that complies with the ACA Code of Ethics and NAADAC guidelines.

Taylor has been meeting with Client B via TMH for about two months. Client B has a diagnosis of opioid use disorder, moderate, in early remission (*DSM-5-TR*, F11.21), and is on maintenance therapy. Client B is prescribed buprenorphine, specifically suboxone, as a component of their medication-assisted treatment. Client B provides a toxicology sample at an off-site lab about once a month. Client B has legal concerns related to their substance use and is a part of a court-ordered drug treatment program. Taylor must report any deviations from scheduled treatment or return to use to Client B's probation officer. Client B's URICA results during intake indicated they were in the action phase of recovery, having recently completed a 30-day inpatient program before transferring to the outpatient center.

During their weekly TMH video session, Taylor notices that Client B's pupils appear constricted (e.g., miosis) and that Client B struggles to stay awake and engaged. Taylor respectfully confronts Client B, pointing out these observations and asking Client B when the last time was that they used opioids. Client B states that they haven't used at all and are just tired because they worked an overnight shift, but also repositions themselves away from the camera. Taylor follows up by asking Client B about their MAT treatment and how they are feeling on the suboxone. Client B reports that "it's not going so great right now because I tried to help a friend out who was struggling and gave them a few strips. I've been cutting mine in half and quarters to try and get to my next appointment."

Questions

1. Assuming good intentions, what did Taylor do well?
2. What ethical issues were you aware of when reading the case? Consider both those that were adhered to and those that were possible risks.
3. What are your thoughts and feelings on using TMH with Client B, based on their stage of recovery and treatment plan?
4. What are your thoughts and feelings on using TMH in combination with Client B receiving MAT? Do you see any risks or benefits to this client's combined TMH/MAT treatment?
5. If you were Taylor, what would be your next steps in this session and following the case? Does Client B's involvement in a court-mandated treatment program influence your considerations or next steps?

Discussion

1. Students review the case at the beginning of the lesson. The instructor may allow students to research the items in the case, such as suboxone or URICA results.
2. Students can discuss the review questions above as a class, in pairs, or small groups, and share their responses with the class. Online asynchronous classes may wish to use discussion boards to share their thoughts on the case.
3. The instructor can summarize the class's primary beliefs about TMH and addictions counseling, placing them into three categories: 1) Benefits, 2) Risks, and 3) Suggestions.

Assessment of Objectives

Assessment of the lesson objectives can be conducted formally or informally. Informal assessment would involve group discussion via in-person or synchronous classes or online discussion boards for asynchronous classes. Instructors can adapt the assignment to a written paper, where students review the case and provide a summary of the discussion questions.

12

Career Counseling

Chapter 6 differentiated between career services and career counseling (NCDA, 2024) and the importance of that distinction when providing telemental health (TMH) services. Career counseling has a unique role that combines personal counseling and career development services. The importance of career development is embedded in the CACREP Foundational Counseling Curriculum, as evidenced by Section 3.D (Career Development). In addition, CACREP recognizes career counseling as a stand-alone profession and master's degree, distinct from other specializations with which it regularly overlaps, such as school counseling or college/student affairs counseling.

Key Concepts

CACREP Standards

CACREP Standards Section 5.B (Career Counseling) outlines eight learning outcomes related to Career Counseling. Table 12.1 provides examples of how TMH can be infused into career counseling curricular training. If these concepts are unfamiliar, the instructor is encouraged to explore the training and reading materials suggested in Chapter 1.

Table 12.1

CACREP Section 5.B (Career Counseling) and Suggested TMH Content

CACREP Standards (2024)	Suggested TMH Content
5.B.1. Factors that affect clients' attitudes toward work and their career decision-making processes.	Capacity for exploring client histories and attitudes to overlap with personal counseling, and the need to maintain a professional role within the scope of practice for TMH delivery; strategies to assess attitudes and decision-making processes (e.g., standardized assessments, checklists, card sorts) and adapting those assessments to TMH delivery (see Chapter 9).
5.B.2. The unique needs and characteristics of diverse clients with regard to career exploration, employment expectations, and socioeconomic issues.	Consideration of cultural and socioeconomic factors in TMH delivery (see Chapter 4); awareness of varied employment trends and employment prospects in different geographic locations where TMH career counseling is provided.
5.B.3. Implications of gender roles and responsibilities for employment, education, family, and leisure	Conducting career intake interviews via TMH, including career history, capacity for personal history, to blur boundaries with career needs—TMH restrictions based on certification and license (see Chapter 6).
5.B.4. Impact of globalization on careers and the workplace.	The capacity for TMH and the internet to connect clients and counselors to vast information on a global scale, as well as the risks and benefits of providing TMH career counseling to clients in different countries beyond the U.S.

CACREP Standards (2024)	Suggested TMH Content
5.B.5. Education, training, employment trends, and labor market information and resources that provide information about job tasks, functions, salaries, requirements, and future outlooks related to broad occupational fields and individual occupations.	Use of online career development tools (e.g., Department of Labor, Bureau of Labor Statistics, *Occupational Outlook Handbook* (OOH), O*Net) and using these tools remotely with clients (see Chapter 6).
5.B.6. Approaches and resources relevant to diverse clients acquiring a set of career planning, employability, job search, job creation, and life-work role transition skills.	Consideration of cultural and SES factors in TMH delivery (see Chapter 4); use of resources for diverse populations in TMH settings (e.g., *My Next Move in Spanish*, Job Accommodations Network, translation services)—practice using these tools with diverse clients via TMH delivery.
5.B.7. Strategies to assist clients in the appropriate use of technology for career information and planning.	Chapter 6: Expanse of career information online, including career assessments and strategies to utilize these tools in TMH delivery; benefit of using various modalities for career counseling (e.g., email, video).
5.B.8. Strategies to market and promote career counseling resources and services	Making clear distinctions about the services provided, specifically if practicing via TMH and across state lines, clarify the counselor's qualification and referral policies as needed.

Career Counseling Is Professional Counseling

Counselors-in-training (CITs) learning to be career counselors recognize that career counseling is considered professional counseling. In Chapter 6, I reviewed the NCDA Code of Ethics definition for *career counseling* (NCDA, 2024, p. 3), including its emphasis on the capacity for career counseling to occur at a deeper level and to address personal/social concerns. As such, instructors must emphasize the potential for blurred lines between career and personal issues. When a client's primary issue is focused on a personal concern instead of a career concern, a career counselor may or may not be qualified to address those concerns, depending on their scope of practice and licensing.

Since practice and licensing laws for professional counseling vary from state to state (see Chapter 3), the use of TMH in these settings could be subject to licensing laws from multiple states.

AI and Career Development

Artificial intelligence (AI) is used in many facets of society. From the use of ChatGPT to AI-generated photos, videos, and images, AI has become common in settings such as education and work. In both career counseling and career development services, clients seek assistance with career advancement tasks such as writing resumes, cover letters, writing samples for jobs, or essays to support their college application, and developing tools such as portfolios. The use of AI to support these projects may be common and appealing to clients and students, yet career counselors need to address both the benefits and risks of using AI to support their career and educational goals. The use of AI in career counseling and development is not specific to TMH delivery but is worthy of attention when discussing technology and career services.

The use of AI has become so common that many organizations have developed policies around its use and require disclosures when AI has been used. Instructors can help CITs learn to research AI policies, and CITs can practice providing psychoeducation to clients on the use of AI in career counseling. Similarly, clients should be aware of when they may consume AI content through basic internet searches. While AI provides many benefits, one of the challenges is identifying the source of information that is gathered, collected, and displayed. When using information for career or education purposes, clients want to be sure that information is both accurate and honest. When delivering services via TMH, the use of screen-sharing video features can support psychoeducation and career counseling interventions.

Teaching Techniques

Instructors can incorporate TMH into the career counseling curriculum for CITs in a variety of ways. Below is a list of suggested strategies that might reinforce or supplement CITs' understanding of TMH and career counseling. These strategies utilize andragogical principles, including self-motivated learning, using prior experiences, recognizing a need for information, and immediately applying learning in a real-world context (Knowles, 1975).

1. *Comparing the NCDA, NECA, and ACA Codes of Ethics.* Chapter 6 addresses the ACA and NCDA Codes of Ethics, as well as NECA's guidance to follow the ACA Code. CITs can examine these codes for variations and similarities, particularly in reference to career services and career counseling and the unique elements of each role regarding TMH.
2. *Examining Career Services and Career Counseling.* NCDA stresses the importance of defining the roles of career counseling and career services in order to engage in ethical practice. CITs can examine various career positions by looking at job openings or exploring the roles of professionals in career centers. Examine the duties of each position to determine which fall into the realm of career counseling and which fall into career services. CITs and instructors can discuss the ethics of using TMH in these real-world positions, particularly the need for licensure to practice TMH in these capacities.
3. *Career Counseling Intakes.* Consider various career counseling intake approaches, such as the Career Construction Interview (Savickas & Hartung, 2012). CITs can practice administering these interventions via TMH and critique the strengths and challenges of conducting a career counseling intake via TMH.
4. *Career Assessments: Counseling or Services?* In Chapter 6, one teaching technique instructed CITs to practice providing Career Assessments in face-to-face (F2F) and TMH settings. In this activity, career CIT can examine those same online assessments to determine if the assessment's purpose, results, and administration would classify as career counseling or career services. Using information from Chapters 6 and 9, CITs can explore the reliability and validity of using these instruments in TMH settings.
5. *Exploring Career Counseling and Career Services Cases.* Many instructors use cases to teach career development and career counseling (recommended resources include Niles et al., 2013). CITs can examine cases from both a career counseling and a career services lens, identifying which case elements would require which interventions. CITs can examine services for these cases in both F2F and TMH delivery and additional precautions and protocols needed for TMH delivery.
6. *Representing Counseling Credentials Accurately.* Chapters 6 and 12 address the importance of accurately representing counseling

skills and credentials when providing TMH career services, particularly across state lines. CITs can practice writing a statement that would be used to represent their services and credentials on their marketing materials. These statements would include clarification of their counseling credentials, training in TMH, services, and connection to relevant state licensing boards, or professional development organizations.

7. *Career Counseling Transitioning to Mental Health Needs.* At times, clients will come for career counseling when other mental health issues are present. Some examples include mental illness, addiction, or personality characteristics that have impacted their ability to be successful in the workplace. CITs and instructors can discuss the challenges of identifying mental health needs when delivering TMH services and the need to make referrals for issues beyond their scope of practice. CITs can role-play addressing their concerns with the client during TMH mock sessions and broaching potential referral needs.
8. *Researching Distance Referral Sources.* TMH services may not be appropriate for all clients; when not, a referral must be made (ACA, 2014; NCDA, 2024). Instructors can lead CITs in an activity where they research referral sources for career concerns and mental health needs in remote/distance areas. CITs can share their strategies for identifying reputable referral sources and vetting these sources before referral.
9. *ChatGPT/AI and Writing.* Instructors and CITs should take time to explore ChatGPT and AI resources that support professional writing, such as cover letters, resumes, writing samples, and college essays. CITs should be familiar with the strengths and pitfalls of these tools and any policies that might accompany their use. CITs can create "pros/cons" lists on AI use in career services and practice using psychoeducation to discuss the list with clients.
10. *Career Development Teaching Techniques.* Instructors can revisit the 10 teaching techniques discussed in Chapter 6 on Career Development and apply them to career counseling instruction.

Sample Lesson: Exploring Values in the Career Decision-Making Process via TMH

James Bethea, PhD, LMHC, CRC
St. John's University

Lesson Objective

At the end of this lesson, graduate students in counseling will be able to facilitate a distance career development activity with young adults (grades 9–12 or undergraduate students) to help students identify, define, and prioritize job values.

2024 CACREP Standards

Standard 3.D.5 (Strategies for assessing abilities, interests, values, personality, and other factors that contribute to career development).

Materials and/or Technology Required

Values Checklist and Reflection Questions (included in the lesson). These items can be sent via email or posted to the learning management system (e.g., Blackboard, Canvas, Google Classroom) for students engaging in online instruction.

Estimated Time Required for Lesson Delivery

45–60 minutes.

Structure and Audience for Lesson

Whole class or small group discussion; the lesson can be delivered via live classroom instruction, online synchronous instruction, or asynchronously via discussion boards.

Lesson Content and Instructional Strategies

1. The instructor will begin the discussion by providing a brief overview of Duane Brown's values-based theory, highlighting values' importance in career choice. According to Brown (2016), satisfaction with a job can be predicted based on how one's values align with a specific work environment. The instructor can

vary the delivery of this information depending on the format of class instruction.

2. The instructor will introduce the Work Values Worksheet (following the lesson) and have students identify and rank their top 10 values from the list provided or include a value(s) not on the checklist. Students will then be asked to select their top 5 core values (from the list of 10) and operationalize them as the meaning of the values may vary across participants. This form can be adapted to digital formats. The instructor models how to facilitate this activity during a live, synchronous lesson or can have students practice administering this checklist during group or individual TMH sessions. The instructor and CITs can also discuss how this activity could be facilitated during asynchronous counseling sessions, including email or chat.
3. Finally, the instructor will pose reflection questions for the students to complete and discuss (listed at the end of this lesson). The instructor can model this facilitation when delivering TMH career counseling in both synchronous (video or phone) and asynchronous (email or chat) sessions.
4. After completing this exercise, students will discuss the strengths and challenges of delivering this career development lesson via distance counseling to students at different developmental levels (e.g., high school, college, etc.).
5. Working in groups, pairs, or individually, students will brainstorm, discuss, and share strategies for delivering the lesson to clients and students in a distance format. Students can also discuss the propensity for career values to intersect with personal values and the importance of clarifying the career counselor role when providing TMH services.

Assessment of Objective

At the end of the lesson, students will present their strategies for delivering the career values lesson via distance technology.

References

Brown, D. (2016). Career information, career counseling, and career development. Pearson.

Work Values Worksheet and Work Values Discussion Questions

Work Values Worksheet

What is important to you in a career? What do you value? What do you believe in? ______________________________

____

Please rank, in order, the 10 career values that are most important to you (with 1 being the most important) from the list below:

Working with people

Rapid advancement

Job security

Working with things

Routine activity

High salary

Independence

Creativity

Power

Flexible work schedule

See results of work

Travel with work

Prestigious title

Routine schedule

Being a team member

Working hands-on

Problem-solving

Ability to structure one's work

Work outdoors

Freedom to express ideas

Improve others' quality of life.

Other:

Other:

Other:

Now that you've examined and prioritized your chosen values and rated them according to their importance, it is time to narrow down those most important to you. For the final step of this exercise, narrow your list of 10 values to your 5 highest priority values. Think of these core values as those that you absolutely would not be able to work without. Please list and operationalize (describe) them below in the space provided in order, with 1 being your highest priority value:

Value	Description
1.	
2.	
3.	
4.	
5.	

Congratulations! You now have a list of your core workplace values representing who you are and what you find most important about work. These core values will likely determine your satisfaction level in your chosen career field.

Work Values Reflection Questions

As you look to the future and consider how you might use this information when choosing a major or career path, use the following questions to guide your reflection and record your responses below:

- What event or experience helped you understand these values were important to you? Consider reflecting on the events or experiences that led to your selecting each of your core values.
- How well do your core values complement the major or job titles you are considering pursuing?
- Will the work that is a part of this major (or the work that is a part of this job) allow you to express the things most important to you? Expand on how your values and intended major and career path match well with your core values.
- What might be missing from the major or job you are considering? In other words, will this major or job NOT allow you to express one of your core values?

Once you have a clear picture of what you really value, it will be easier to identify careers that complement those values. If you have a position that conflicts with your values, you will not be happy and generally will enjoy less success in that position over the long term. Content in the worksheet was retrieved from the following websites: https://www.ndm.edu and https://www.winona.edu.

Sample Lesson: Asynchronous Career Counseling - Case Study, Questions, and Discussion

Heather C. Robertson, PhD, LMHC, CRC, NCC, BC-TMH
St. John's University

Lesson Objectives

At the end of this lesson, students will have

1) examined a case using asynchronous career counseling,
2) applied concepts learned in the program to the case, and
3) decided on an ethical course of action regarding the case.

2024 CACREP Standards

Standard 5.B.7 (Strategies to assist clients in the appropriate use of technology for career information and planning).

Materials and/or Technology Required

Access to case study.

Preparation Required

Prior instruction on TMH career counseling and ethical codes.

Estimated Time Required for Lesson Delivery

This activity should last approximately 30–45 minutes, depending on instructional time.

Structure and Audience for Lesson

This activity is best used in master's level counselor training in career counseling. Format can be in-person or online (synchronous or asynchronous).

Lesson Content and Instructional Strategies

Case Example

Aiden is a career counselor who manages their own distance career counseling practice. The website for their company, ACC, specifies that their role is to provide career development services, not career counseling. The website specifies that they provide asynchronous services via email, including resume and cover letter reviews, job search skills, interview skills, and salary negotiation strategies. Their credentials are listed as having a master's degree in career counseling and a certification as a Global Career Development Facilitator (GCDF) with links to the Center for Credentialing and Education (CCE) website. They publish rates on the website for each of the services provided. To save costs, Aiden uses a free email service for their business.

Client C emails Aiden for help with a resume and job search:

> "Dear Aiden, I found your website, and I would like some help with my resume and job search. I am not currently working but I will find a way to pay the fees posted of $100 for resume review and $200 for job search assistance. I need a resume to start my job search and I don't have one. I have not been working due to caring for my children and my aging parents. I hope to work full-time since I really need the money. I am recently divorced and have a lot of expenses. I have not worked in an office, but I would like to do office work because I have good computer skills. Working remotely would be best for me. I previously worked in retail. Hope that you can help me. Sincerely, Client C."

Aiden receives the email and believes they will be able to help Client C. Aiden replies:

> "Dear Client C, thank you for your email, and I look forward to working with you. Attached, please find a link to the payment information where you can pay for the resume review. Since you don't already have a resume, it would be $150 for resume development. Once the fee

is paid, I will send you a draft resume within a week, or I will return your resume with a review within a week of receiving it. I need more information to assist you with your job search. Please complete this attached questionnaire, which includes your work history, the geographic preferences for your work, as well as a work values, interests, and skills survey. Please email that form back to me for next steps, along with payment, and we will begin on the job search strategy work. Looking forward to working with you. Sincerely, Aiden."

Questions

1. Assuming good intentions, what did Aiden do well? Consider their actions in both establishing their business and their email interactions.
2. What ethical issues were you aware of when reading the case? Consider both those that were adhered to and those that were possible risks.
3. What thoughts, concerns, or questions do you have about using asynchronous career counseling? Do you think asynchronous counseling is appropriate for Client C? What else needs to be considered in asynchronous TMH counseling as opposed to synchronous TMH counseling?
4. What thoughts, concerns, or questions do you have about Client C's personal needs versus career counseling needs?
5. What other thoughts, questions, concerns, or suggestions do you have regarding this case?

Discussion

1. Students review the case at the beginning of the lesson.
2. Students discuss the review questions above as a class, in pairs, or in small groups, and share their responses with the class. Online asynchronous classes may wish to use discussion boards to share their thoughts on the case.
3. The instructor can summarize the class's primary beliefs and place them into three categories: 1) did well, 2) did not do well, and 3) Suggestions. This model allows students to recognize that counselors rarely act maliciously and often do many things well,

even if they make mistakes. Students may also offer alternative suggestions that Aiden could have used.

Assessment of Objectives

Informal assessments involve group discussion via in-person, synchronous classes, or asynchronous online discussion boards. Formal assessments can include a written paper, where students review the case, research the assessments, and provide a written summary of areas in which Aiden 1) did well, 2) did not do well, and 3) suggestions.

13

Clinical Mental Health Counseling

Clinical mental health counseling (CMHC) is recognized as a specialization within the counseling profession. The importance of understanding mental health, mental illness, crisis, and trauma is embedded in Section 3 (Foundational Counseling Curriculum) of the 2024 CACREP Standards. These concepts are addressed by the following standards:

- 3.C.12: The influence of mental and physical health conditions on coping, resilience, and overall wellness for individuals and families across the lifespan.
- 3.C.13: Effects of crises, disasters, stress, grief, and trauma across the lifespan.
- 3.E.18: Classification, effects, and indications of commonly prescribed psychopharmacological medications.
- 3.E.19: Suicide prevention and response models and strategies.
- 3.E.20: Crisis intervention, trauma-informed, community-based, and disaster mental health strategies.
- 3.G.10: Use of structured interviewing, symptom checklists, and personality and psychological testing.
- 3.G.11: Diagnostic processes, including differential diagnosis and the use of current diagnostic classification systems.

- 3.G.13: Procedures for assessing and responding to risk of aggression or danger to others, self-inflicted harm, and suicide.

Thus, even students not specializing in CMHC will receive some foundational knowledge in mental health concepts. In addition to these general concepts, CACREP recognizes CMHC as a stand-alone profession, distinct from other specializations.

The American Mental Health Counselors Association (AMHCA) updated its Code of Ethics in 2020, specifically Section B.6 (The Use of Technology-Supported Counseling and Communications [TSCC]). AMHCA standards recognize diverse telemental health (TMH) modalities in Item 5.6.a. where they define TSCC as "a medium to counseling (e.g., providing services via phone, text, video, etc.)" (p. 6). AMHCA requires counselors to receive training (5.6.d) before delivering TMH services, and counselors must collect emergency contact information at the beginning of TMH services (5.6.f). Instructors are charged with training CMHC counselors-in-training (CMHC-CITs) in TMH, particularly in identifying emergency resources.

Key Concepts

CACREP Standards

CACREP Standards Section 5.C (Clinical Mental Health Counseling) outlines nine learning outcomes related to CMHC counseling. These standards do not specifically address the use of TMH delivery. However, there are distinct and discernable connections to content on TMH in the CMHC curriculum, as outlined in Table 13.1. If suggested concepts are unfamiliar, the instructor is encouraged to explore the training and reading materials suggested in Chapter 1.

Table 13.1

CACREP Section 5.C (Clinical Mental Health Counseling) and Suggested TMH Content

CACREP Standards (2024)	Suggested TMH Content
5.C.1. Etiology, nomenclature, diagnosis, treatment, referral, and prevention of mental, behavioral, and neurodevelopmental disorders.	Exploring treatment, referral, and prevention strategies if/when using TMH. Selecting appropriate TMH services in relation to mental health, behavioral, and neurodevelopmental needs.

CACREP Standards (2024)	Suggested TMH Content
5.C.2. Mental health service delivery modalities and networks within the continuum of care, such as primary care, outpatient, partial treatment, inpatient, integrated behavioral healthcare, and aftercare.	Use of TMH with different levels of care, e.g., providing TMH for outpatient care versus using TMH for collateral or behavioral health integration for inpatient care (Schaffer et al., 2020).
5.C.3. Legislation, government policy, and regulatory processes relevant to clinical mental health counseling.	Importance of advocacy for the CMHC profession and for client access to both mental health care and digital tools. Licensing guidelines in various states (Epstein Becker Green, 2024) and the Counseling Compact. Access to mental health care improved via TMH (e.g., Counseling Compact) only with digital access (see Chapter 4).
5.C.4. Intake interview, mental status evaluation, biopsychosocial history, mental health history, and psychological assessment for treatment planning and caseload management.	Challenges when using TMH (e.g., video, phone) for mental health intake, mental status exam, and assessment (e.g., sensory limitations); benefit of TMH to connect people to services, assessment, evaluation, and resources, such as psychiatric services (Alicata et al., 2016; Glover et al., 2013; Hilty et al., 2015; Hoffman & Kane, 2013; Pullen et al., 2013; Sunderji et al., 2014).
5.C.5. Techniques and interventions for prevention and treatment of a broad range of mental health issues.	Selection and use of TMH for different clients based on mental health issues, development, technological skills, and digital access (see literature below on various mental health conditions and the use of TMH).
5.C.6. Strategies for interfacing with the legal system regarding court-referred clients.	Encryption and security of transmitting and communicating court-ordered reports via secure technology

CACREP Standards (2024)	Suggested TMH Content
5.C.7. Strategies for interfacing with integrated behavioral health care professionals.	Benefit of TMH to increase access to a wide range of behavioral health providers (e.g., collateral contacts, medical providers); risks of information security and confidentiality transmitting TMH data to outside providers.
5.C.8. Strategies to advocate for people with mental, behavioral, and neurodevelopmental conditions.	Advocacy efforts to include access to technological and mental health resources; using TMH to increase access is only possible with advocacy to reduce the digital divide.
5.C.9. Third-party reimbursement and other practice and management issues in clinical mental health counseling.	Insurance, Medicaid, and Medicare reimbursement models for TMH treatment (Luxton et al., 2023); restrictions to reimbursement and/or state funding for TMH service delivery; use of EMR and data security.

Mental Health Advocacy and TMH Treatment

One area that instructors can reinforce is the importance of advocacy for access to mental health treatment. CMHC-CITs and all professional counselors are responsible for advocating for our profession and our clients. CMHC can advocate for increased access to mental health counseling services, including TMH counseling services. In Chapter 4, I discussed health professional shortage areas (HPSA), the digital divide, and the Counseling Compact. Instructors training CITs in CMHC TMH practice can advise students on advocacy issues, including mental health care and technology access.

The effective use of TMH with mental health disorders is well documented in professional literature, including posttraumatic stress disorder (PTSD; Acierno et al., 2016; Weiss et al., 2018), anxiety disorders (Arnberg et al., 2014; Carpenter et al., 2018), and depression (Forsell et al., 2017; Hobbs et al., 2018), as well as severe mental illness (SMI) (Lawes-Wickar et al., 2018; Medalia et al., 2020; Miu et al., 2020). CMHC uses many of the TMH concepts discussed elsewhere in this book, such as counseling communication (Chapter 7), group dynamics (Chapter 8), and assessment and diagnosis (Chapter 9). Thus, instructors training CMHC-CITs can reference earlier resources to support their instruction.

Safety Planning in TMH Mental Health Treatment

One of the challenges discussed in Chapter 7 is managing TMH emergency situations from a distance. This includes collecting emergency contact information, informed consent, verifying the client's location, and identifying nearby emergency facilities. For CMHC, one of the counselor's primary roles may be creating safety plans with clients who have thoughts of suicide or homicide. Instructors can help CITs practice TMH safety planning in their training programs while exposing them to various TMH tools used for safety planning.

There are a variety of strategies and tools used in safety planning. One strategy is verbally articulating and discussing a safety plan with a client, which can be used in both face-to-face (F2F) and TMH sessions. This strategy can be as simple as reiterating the use of #988, crisis phone lines and text services, or detailing a plan of action for support. When using asynchronous TMH counseling, the benefit of typing or texting a safety plan is that it creates a written record for the client, yet there is also a risk of maintaining the security of that information. For TMH synchronous video sessions, written safety plans can be reviewed on a shared screen and emailed to both parties for their record. More recently, safety planning mobile apps have emerged. Unlike verbal or written plans on a shared screen, it may be more difficult for a CMHC provider to confirm the use of these apps and content unless the client can show/share the screen with the counselor. Some apps allow for sharing safety plans with others and may also notify designees when plans have been edited. A CMHC provider who requests or requires that a client include them on their safety plan app will want to explore the legal and ethical issues involved and the security and encryption standards of these tools. CMHC providers should not recommend mobile apps that have not been vetted and deemed appropriate for client use.

Teaching Techniques

Instructors can provide instruction on TMH to CMHC-CITs in various ways. Below is a list of suggested strategies to reinforce or supplement instruction of TMH CMHC practice. These strategies utilize andragogical principles, including self-motivated learning, using prior experiences, recognizing a need for information, and immediately applying learning in a real-world context (Knowles, 1975).

1. *Reviewing Mental Health TMH Counseling Ethics.* CITs should begin with a review/refresher of counseling ethical codes that pertain

to research and TMH. These include the ACA Code of Ethics (2024) Section H (Distance Counseling) and AMHCA Standard B.6 (The Use of Technology-Supported Counseling and Communications). The instructor and CITs can explore areas where the codes are complementary and conflicting in relation to TMH and CMHC.

2. *Mental Status Exam.* CMHC providers regularly complete a mental status exam (MSE) as a part of their intake and assessment procedures. Instructors can have CITs review sample MSEs and explore challenges to gathering MSE information in a TMH session. Consider all modalities of TMH (e.g., video, phone) and the need for counselor observation during the MSE.
3. *Diagnostic Criteria and Limited Senses.* As instructors teach psychopathology and DSM criteria, pause to explore with CITs how using TMH might impact the observation, reporting, and/or recording of these criteria. How might identifying the criteria be affected by the counselor's limited senses? Consider all TMH Modalities, as well as a variety of mental health disorders, including disorders diagnosed in children.
4. *Co-occurring Disorders.* CMHC providers are aware of the propensity of mental health disorders to co-occur with substance use disorders (SUD). Instructors can utilize information from Chapter 11 to help CMHC-CITs explore how they might encounter SUD in their work and strategies they may need to employ to assess and treat SUD concurrently with mental illness.
5. *Safety Planning via Multiple Modalities.* CITs can practice conducting a safety plan with clients using multiple TMH modalities. CITs can engage in mock sessions to conduct safety planning via video, phone, email, and chat. Instructors can help CITs explore the benefits and risks of conducting safety planning in multiple TMH modalities.
6. *Safety Planning Apps.* Safety planning mobile apps are becoming more common. CMHCs need to be comfortable using these tools and teaching their clients how to use them. Instructors can advise CITs to explore various apps and practice creating safety plans. CITs can also practice introducing a safety planning app to clients and describing its use.
7. *Mobile App Security.* Mobile apps that are recommended to clients, including safety planning apps, must be vetted by counselors to be appropriate and clinically sound. Other examples include mindfulness apps and symptom-tracking apps. The American

Psychiatric Association "App Advisor" provides a checklist for counselors when considering mobile apps (APA, 2024). Instructors can advise CITs to select and evaluate a safety planning app using the App Advisor. Remind students that apps update regularly and may need to be reevaluated in the future. CITs can report their findings to the class.

8. *Minors and Mental Health.* Consider the use of mental health treatment with minors. What elements would need to be changed or enhanced if TMH is provided? Consider the different developmental levels of the client (e.g., child, adolescent), as well as the presenting issue (e.g., developmental, behavioral, social/emotional) and the modality (e.g., video, phone). Consider procedural changes (e.g., informed consent), changes to clinical interventions, and parent involvement.
9. *Collaborative Care.* Mental health treatment often requires collaborative care between the counselor, service providers, and medical professionals, as well as collateral support from family. Instructors and CITs can explore how TMH can be both a risk and a benefit to collaborative care models. Consider issues of access, security, and different TMH modalities.
10. *Continuum of Care.* CMHC is delivered in various settings, including primary care, outpatient, partial treatment, inpatient, integrated behavioral health care, and aftercare. Instructors and CITs can explore the risks and benefits of using TMH in different treatment settings. Consider issues of access, security, and different TMH modalities.

Sample Lesson: Diagnosis and Treatment Planning via Telemental Health

Robert Eschenauer, PhD, LMHC, NCC
St. John's University

Lesson Objectives

At the end of this lesson, students will have

1) examined DSM-5-TR criteria for diagnostic symptoms,
2) discussed the potential treatment interventions for specific diagnoses, and

3) explored the impact of using TMH to collect diagnostic information and develop a treatment plan.

2024 CACREP Standards

Standards 3.G.11 (Diagnostic processes, including differential diagnosis and the use of current diagnostic classification systems), 5.C.4 (Intake interview, mental status evaluation, biopsychosocial history, mental health history, and psychological assessment for treatment planning and caseload management), and 5.C.5 (Techniques and interventions for the prevention and treatment of a broad range of mental health issues).

Materials or Technology Required

DSM-5-TR; a textbook for treatment planning and diagnosis instruction can also support this lesson.

Preparation Required

Students should have received prior instruction on DSM-5 diagnosis and general treatment planning guidelines. Using content from Chapter 10 of this book, the students have also received instruction on TMH practice in mental health counseling.

Estimated Time Required for Lesson Delivery

Prior instruction time may vary. The time for this activity is approximately 45–60 minutes.

Structure and Audience for Lesson

This activity is designed for in-person or online instruction. The intended audience is master's students enrolled in clinical mental health counseling programs or those learning about diagnosis and treatment planning.

Lesson Content and Instructional Strategies

1. Instruction is provided on psychopathology and diagnostic criteria for mental illness using the *DSM-5-TR*. Use case examples when possible. For example, during the interview and biopsychosocial history, the client describes anxiety that is extreme and seems to negatively impact all areas of functioning, meeting the diagnostic criteria discussed in F41.1 (Generalized Anxiety Disorder).

2. Instruction is provided to develop a client-centered, evidence-based treatment. For example, the treatment plan includes cognitive behavioral therapy using the diagnosis above.
3. Instruction is provided on using TMH in mental health counseling.
4. The instructor assigns/selects a disorder from the DSM-5-TR for students to review. Note: For this activity, students focus on one specific diagnosis (e.g., major depressive disorder, panic disorder, body dysmorphic disorder). Students may work as a group, in small groups, in pairs, or individually to examine one disorder collectively, or be assigned (or select) individual disorders to examine independently.
5. The instructor has students examine the diagnostic criteria in the *DSM-5-TR* for the disorder and respond to the following questions:
   a. How might you assess these criteria if you were conducting an in-person diagnostic intake interview and/or assessment process? Using the example above, how would you determine the degree of anxiety and worry experienced by the client and the time element involved (how long did it last?)? What specific symptoms were present for more days than not for the past six months? How do these symptoms cause clinically significant distress or impairment in social, occupational, or other important areas of functioning?
   b. How would that intake and evaluation process change if you were conducting a TMH intake interview and/or assessment process? What would be limited about the interview, if anything?
   c. What factors, if any, might impact your interview and assessment results when conducting clinical interviews either in person or online? How could your online observation of the client's behavior while they are answering the questions affect the clinical significance of their answers?
6. When students have thoroughly explored and discussed the differences between online and in-person assessment and interview procedures, the instructor will ask students to examine treatment plan outcomes for a person with this diagnosis. For example, in the case above, cognitive behavioral therapy could be used to treat this disorder. An evidence-based approach could include each of the following steps: psychoeducation, self-awareness, cognitive restructuring, relaxation techniques (progressive muscle

relaxation, breathing techniques, guided imagery), systematic desensitization, and exposure therapy.

7. Students should identify 3 to 4 clinical, evidence-based interventions they might utilize with a client with this diagnosis (case studies from the text may help students generate ideas). Based on the treatment options they select, the instructor leads a discussion on the following questions:
   a. What made you select the clinical intervention/treatments you selected?
   b. How might those interventions and treatments delivered during an in-person session vary if they are delivered during a TMH session? How does that impact your selection of intervention, if at all?
   c. How would you assess client progress using these clinical interventions for in-person and telehealth treatment? Using the example above, interviews and rating scales will determine the effectiveness of the techniques. Observing the client when using these techniques in in-person and TMH sessions will let the counselor know if the technique was completed correctly and if it was effective.
   d. What else might you need to consider if you were providing telehealth services to this client instead of in-person? For example, in-person sessions could use electromyography (EMG) feedback to monitor patient progress.
8. At the conclusion of the discussion, the instructor summarizes the group feedback and encourages students to consider both telemental health and in-person treatment options when conducting clinical interviews and creating treatment plans.

Assessment of Objectives

The lesson objectives will be assessed via the classroom discussion and the students' response to the activity. Students may also be asked to reference this activity in a reflective journal of another assignment.

References

American Psychiatric Association. (2022). *Diagnostic and statistical manual of mental disorders 5-TR* (5th ed., text revision.).

Sample/suggested textbooks to supplement lesson

Berman, P.S. (2019). *Case conceptualization and treatment planning: Integrating theory with clinical practice* (4th ed.). Sage.

Schwitzer, A. M., Pope, A. L. & Rubin, L. C. (2024). *Diagnosis and treatment planning skills: A popular culture casebook approach* (3rd ed.). Sage.

Zubernis, L., & Snyder, M. (2016). Case conceptualization and effective interventions. Sage.

Sample Lesson: Identifying Symptoms of Antisocial Personality Disorder (APD)

Jessica L. Sniatecki, PhD, CRC
SUNY Brockport

Lesson Objectives

At the end of this lesson, students will be able to:

1) Identify DSM-5 diagnostic symptoms of antisocial personality disorder (APD) through observation, including limits to observation via TMH.
2) Determine appropriate treatment goals based on reported and observed clinical symptoms and client reports, including limits to observation via TMH.
3) Explore factors that may be sources of strength/growth for the client and consider how these might be capitalized on in treatment to foster success.
4) Demonstrate awareness of how mental health symptoms may impact client experiences, both in treatment and in real-world settings.

2024 CACREP Standards

Standards 3.G.11 (Diagnostic processes, including differential diagnosis and the use of current diagnostic classification systems), 5.C.4 (Intake interview, mental status evaluation, biopsychosocial history, mental health history, and psychological assessment for treatment planning and caseload management), and 5.D.9 (Third-party reimbursement and other practice and management issues in clinical mental health counseling).

Materials and/or Technology Required

If the activity is done in-person, a computer with a projector and speakers is required. Online instruction requires access to audio/video and internet.

Preparation Required

Minimal. The facilitator should review the video clip and prepare guiding questions that are relevant to the audience and setting.

Estimated Time Required for Lesson Delivery

30–60 minutes, depending on the number of participants and their questions/comments (for in-person or synchronous administration).

Structure and Audience for Lesson

This activity can be completed both online and in-person and with a variety of audiences, including both undergraduate and graduate students.

Lesson Content and Instructional Strategies

This activity assists participants in identifying the diagnostic symptoms of APD and exploring how information gleaned in a clinical interview can be incorporated into clinical work with clients. After watching a YouTube clip on APD (https://www.youtube.com/watch?v=_ZYWLpqvgnI [First interview]), participants will identify the specific diagnostic (DSM) symptoms they observed. In this video, the interviewer is face-to-face (F2F) with the client. The instructor and students should discuss how this interview might differ if conducted via TMH, including video or phone.

Next, students are prompted to identify specific treatment goals for the client. The instructor and students should discuss how these interventions might be different if treatment was conducted via TMH, including video, phone, text, or email treatment. Finally, students are asked to identify components of the interview that may constitute "glimmers of hope" and/or areas of strength for this client and identify ways that these might build upon these in clinical work to facilitate progress toward treatment goals. In an F2F setting, the entire group may view the clip together and then break into smaller groups to respond to the prompts and explore ideas. A large-group discussion led by the facilitator can then be used to debrief and summarize what each group discussed and identified in their work together.

This activity can also be administered in an online, asynchronous format for participants to view the video example independently and then respond to the prompts via online discussion or a similar setting. During the discussion, the instructor and students can address how they can utilize these skills when working with clients in a TMH setting or conducting distance intake, assessment, and treatment planning.

Assessment of Objectives

The identified learning objectives are typically accomplished by completing this activity. The facilitator may also formally evaluate learning objectives via exam/quiz questions, written assignments, or other means.

Resources

Video case example: https://www.youtube.com/watch?v=_ZYWLpqvgnI (First interview)

DSM-5-TR diagnostic criteria for APD.

14

Clinical Rehabilitation Counseling

The role of certified rehabilitation counselors (CRCs) is defined by the Commission on Rehabilitation Counselor Certification (CRCC) as having "specialized knowledge, skills, and abilities to collaborate with persons with all types of disabilities to overcome barriers to employment or other life domains" (CRCC, 2023, p. 3). Rehabilitation counselors work with people with disabilities (PWD), with physical, cognitive, sensory, emotional, medical, and mental health disorders. The rehabilitation counselor's role extends beyond employment counseling, yet many CRCs work in vocational rehabilitation counseling settings. Like clinical mental health counselors (CMHCs) and addictions counselors, rehabilitation counselors provide counseling in both face-to-face (F2F) and telemental health (TMH) settings. The term *telerehabilitation* is often used in rehabilitation counseling literature to describe TMH services. While I continue to use "TMH" in this chapter, instructors examining professional literature should consider each of these terms when conducting literature searches.

The Commission on Rehabilitation Education (CORE) previously accredited rehabilitation counseling programs. Following the CACREP/CORE merger, rehabilitation counseling and clinical rehabilitation counseling programs receive accreditation under CACREP. Under the 2024

CACREP standards, Sections 5.D. (Clinical Rehabilitation Counseling) and 5.G (Rehabilitation Counseling) address educational standards for counselors-in-training (CITs). In this chapter, I will address infusing TMH content into both clinical rehabilitation counseling and rehabilitation counseling curricula. Unless otherwise specified, I will use the term *rehabilitation counselor* to include the work of both rehabilitation and clinical rehabilitation counselors.

Key Concepts

CACREP Standards

CACREP Sections 5.D (Clinical Rehabilitation Counseling) and 5.G (Rehabilitation Counseling) include educational standards for counselors-in-training (CITs). While both rehabilitation counseling and clinical rehabilitation counselors provide counseling to PWD, there are distinct differences between the two, including how an instructor can infuse content on TMH into the curriculum. Tables 14.1 and 14.2 provide suggestions on how TMH content can be connected to CACREP standards. If these concepts are unfamiliar, the instructor is reminded to explore the training and reading materials suggested in Chapter 1.

Table 14.1

CACREP Section 5.D (Clinical Rehabilitation Counseling) and Suggested TMH Content

CACREP Standards (2024)	Suggested TMH Content
5.D.1. Effects of the onset, progression, and expected duration of disability on clients' holistic functioning.	Importance of understanding the client's developmental and functional ability to use technology before using TMH services (Froehlich et al., 2023; Holmes et al., 2018).
5.D.2. Environmental, attitudinal, and individual barriers for people with disabilities.	Capacity for TMH to reduce some environmental barriers (e.g., transportation and travel access) and increase access to expanded rehabilitation services for PWD (e.g., multilingual client needs, American Sign Language).

CACREP Standards (2024)	Suggested TMH Content
5.D.3. Impact of disability on sexuality.	Counselor awareness of technology available to support sexuality for PWD and those without (e.g., digisexuality, teledildonics, and AImorosexuality; TMH or F2F delivery; see Chapter 4).
5.D.4. Rehabilitation service delivery systems, including housing, independent living, case management, public benefits programs, educational programs, and public/proprietary vocational rehabilitation programs.	Pros and cons of TMH service delivery for these services, including the ability to participate in interviews (e.g., housing, benefits), accessing services (e.g., education and vocational programs, case management); challenges in delivering on-site services via TMH (e.g., workplace vocational evaluation) (Dorstyn et al., 2022).
5.D.5. Clinical rehabilitation counseling services within the continuum of care, such as inpatient, outpatient, partial hospitalization and aftercare, integrated behavioral health care, and rehabilitation counseling services networks.	Use of TMH with different levels of care along the continuum, e.g., providing TMH for outpatient care vs. using TMH for collateral or behavioral health integration for inpatient care; capacity for TMH to increase collaborative care (Pogoda et al., 2021).
5.D.6. Transferable skills, functional assessments, and work-related supports for achieving and maintaining meaningful employment for people with disabilities.	Challenges of functional assessments utilizing TMH, including limited workplace observations (Holmes et al., 2018).
5.D.7. Role of family, social networks, and community in the provision of services for and treatment of people with disabilities.	Capacity for TMH to support collateral care and integrated support; need for family access to technology for TMH services.
5.D.8. Assistive technology to reduce or eliminate barriers and functional limitations.	TMH technology must accommodate the use of AT devices if needed to access care (Rehabilitation Engineering and Assistive Technology Society of North America [RESNA], 2024).

CACREP Standards (2024)	Suggested TMH Content
5.D.9. Intake interview, mental status evaluation, biopsychosocial history, mental health history, and psychological assessment for treatment planning and caseload management for people with disabilities.	Challenges when using TMH modalities (e.g., video, phone) for intake and assessment (e.g., sensory limitations—see Chapter 9); need for accessible technology, compliant with the Americans with Disabilities Act (ADA; see below).
5.D.10. Strategies to advocate for people with disabilities related to accessibility, accommodations, and disability law adherence.	Advocacy efforts to include access to technological and disability resources; using TMH to increase access only possible with advocacy to reduce the digital divide.
5.D.11. Third-party reimbursement and other practice and management issues in clinical rehabilitation counseling.	Insurance, Medicaid, and Medicare reimbursement models for TMH treatment; restrictions to reimbursement and/or state funding for TMH rehabilitation service delivery; EMR and data security.

Table 14.2

CACREP Section 5.G (Rehabilitation Counseling) and Suggested TMH Content

CACREP Standards 2024	Suggested TMH Related Content
5.G.1. Individual response to disability, including the role of families, communities, and other social networks.	Need to understand the client's disability before using TMH, including client access, support systems, and community resources (Froehlich et al., 2023; Holmes et al., 2018).
5.G.2. Strategies to enhance adjustment and adaptation to disability.	Capacity for TMH to connect PWD to role models, peers, and mentors with diverse disabilities.
5.G.3. Effects of socioeconomic trends, public policies, stigma, access, and attitudinal barriers as they relate to disability.	Instruction on TMH history and increased use of technology, creating additional access to rehabilitation services (if accessible).

CACREP Standards 2024	Suggested TMH Related Content
5.G.4. Principles of independent living, self-determination, and informed choice.	Role of technology (e.g., assistive technology) in increasing client independence and self-determination (TMH or F2F delivery).
5.G.5. Rehabilitation counseling services and organizational settings, including independent living, community rehabilitation, and public/proprietary vocational rehabilitation programs.	Exploring the use of TMH rehabilitation services in different settings (e.g., housing, employment). Selecting appropriate TMH intervention in relation to client, disability, and access needs (Dorstyn et al., 2022).
5.G.6. Benefit systems used by individuals with disabilities, including but not limited to Social Security, governmental monetary assistance, workers' compensation insurance, long-term disability insurance, and veterans' benefits.	Capacity for TMH to enhance access to some services (e.g., housing interviews, benefits interviews). Expanse of benefits information online. Capacity for less human contact (e.g., troubleshooting problems) and capacity for fraud/data risk with online services.
5.G.7. Classification, terminology, etiology, functional capacity, and prognosis of disabilities.	Selection and use of TMH for different clients based on disability, development, technological skills, and digital access.
5.G.8. Career- and work-related assessments, including job analysis, worksite modification, transferable skills analysis, job readiness, and work hardening.	Traditional challenges of TMH Assessment (see Chapter 9), supplemented by challenges in conducting virtual comprehensive vocational evaluations.
5.G.9. Evaluation and application of assistive technology with an emphasis on individualized assessment and planning.	Ensuring successful integration of AT with technological tools used to provide TMH services (RESNA, 2024).
5.G.10. Career development and employment models and strategies for achieving and maintaining meaningful employment for people with disabilities.	Exploring career development models, theories, and interventions for use via TMH with PWD. Considering which models are reliably adapted to TMH and effective with PWD.

CACREP Standards 2024	Suggested TMH Related Content
5.G.11. Strategies to analyze work activity and labor market data and trends to facilitate the match between an individual with a disability and targeted jobs.	Use of online career development tools (e.g., Bureau of Labor Statistics, Department of Labor, OOH, O*Net) and using these tools remotely with clients (see Chapter 6). TMH adaptations for using these tools with PWD.
5.G.12. Case management strategies that facilitate rehabilitation and independent living planning.	Capacity for TMH to increase access to case management services; risks of reducing live visits and observations that typically accompany independent living services (Pogoda et al., 2021).
5.G.13. Consultation and collaboration with employers regarding the legal rights and benefits of hiring individuals with disabilities, including Americans with Disabilities Act adherence, accommodations, universal design, and workplace disability prevention.	Capacity for TMH and virtual consultations to provide access to online information for employers, including ADA resources and job accommodations resources (e.g., Ask JAN); capacity for video sessions to provide visual access to workspaces for rehabilitation counselor recommendations.
5.G.14. Strategies to promote self-advocacy skills of individuals with disabilities.	Exploring how technology training, such as technology utilized for TMH, may increase client self-advocacy skills.
5.G.15. Facilitating client knowledge of and access to community and technology services and resources.	Capacity for rehabilitation counselors to use technology with clients to obtain information on community resources, e.g., public transportation apps for travel training.
5.G.16. Strategies to advocate on behalf of people with disabilities as related to disability and disability legislation.	Advocacy efforts to include access to technological and disability resources.

Access to Counseling

One of the most significant benefits of TMH is access to rehabilitation counseling for PWD. TMH can create access for people with mobility and transportation limitations. It can reduce barriers due to geographic limitations, such as distance and architectural issues (e.g., parking, ramps) or limited access to public transportation. Some medical conditions create obstacles, such as traveling with medical equipment or needing specialized devices. Those accommodations are already in place when providing TMH in the client's home. Some clients with disabilities rely on ride-share services, public transportation, or other costly and unreliable measures of travel, which are eliminated with the use of TMH. Yet, additional barriers may impede TMH engagement and progress. As discussed in Chapter 4, the client must have access to the technology required for TMH treatment, which may be limited by socioeconomic, educational, geographic, or racial factors. PWD who are unemployed may face significant socioeconomic barriers that impede their access to TMH technology.

Research on the use of TMH within rehabilitation counseling varies. In one study, online support groups were used to assist persons who were unemployed or had unstable employment. The study found low engagement, but those who engaged reported higher job-searching activity (Dorstyn et al., 2022). Pogoda et al. (2021) found that Veterans Administration (VA) vocational rehabilitation providers had varied perceptions of TMH delivery. Providers felt TMH increased accessibility and reduced cancellations, but providers preferred in-person sessions. Providers noted challenges with communication, collaboration with the clinical team, and the ability to adapt services to TMH (Pogoda et al., 2021).

Technology Compliance

The primary caution for rehabilitation counselors using TMH is that the technology must be accessible to those receiving services. The Americans with Disabilities Act (ADA), under the division of the U. S. Department of Civil Rights, publishes guidance on web accessibility and the ADA (U.S. Department of Civil Rights, 2022). The guidance provides information on why accessibility matters and examples of barriers to web accessibility (e.g., poor color contrast, lack of alternative text, no captions, mouse-only navigation). The ADA applies to government offices and any business open to the public, including counseling services. They provide information and resources on how to create accessible web information. CITs can review these standards and, if using third-party platforms, assess the accessibility and barriers of the platform.

The use of **assistive technology** (AT) enhances PWD's independence. AT may include text readers or talk-to-text converters for individuals with sensory, motor, or cognitive disabilities. AT can enhance TMH for text-based modalities (e.g., email, chat, text) based on the client's needs, abilities, and preferences. While this AT can be utilized with TMH, rehabilitation counselors must ensure that the technology they use to provide TMH services (e.g., video software) is ADA-compliant and compatible with the AT used by the client.

Teaching Techniques

Instructors can provide instruction on TMH to rehabilitation CITs in various ways. Below is a list of suggested strategies that might reinforce or supplement instruction in TMH rehabilitation practice. These strategies utilize andragogical principles, including self-motivated learning, using prior experiences, recognizing a need for information, and immediately applying learning in a real-world context (Knowles, 1975).

1. *Reviewing Rehabilitation TMH Counseling Ethics.* CITs should begin with a review/refresher of counseling ethical codes that pertain to rehabilitation counseling and TMH. These include the ACA Code of Ethics (2024) Section H (Distance Counseling), as well as the CRCC Code of Ethics (2023) Section K (Technology, Social Media, and Virtual Counseling). The instructor and CITs can explore areas where the codes are complementary and conflicting concerning TMH and rehabilitation counseling.
2. *Americans with Disabilities Act (ADA).* CITs in both rehabilitation counseling and clinical rehabilitation counseling can explore federal laws that impact PWD. Instructors can have CITs take a critical look at the key elements of the ADA and explore the use of TMH as both expanding and limiting access to rehabilitation services.
3. *Web Accessibility.* Instructors can instruct CITs to examine the U.S. Department of Civil Rights guidance on web accessibility. CITs should make note of the key requirements to ensure accessibility. To supplement learning, CITs can critique a website typically used in rehabilitation services and evaluate its web accessibility.
4. *Assistive Technology.* Rehabilitation counselors may be exposed to various types of assistive technology. CIT can explore various types of assistive technology and discuss how they would adapt their TMH practice to support a client using this AT to engage in services. The Assistive Technology Industry Association (ATIA) and the Rehabilitation Engineering and Assistive Technology Society of North America (RESNA) provide information on AT.

5. *Assessment.* CITs in rehabilitation counseling often learn various types of career assessments, from paper-and-pencil to computer-based to workplace evaluations. Instructors can have CITs identify the accommodations needed when providing these career assessments via TMH.
6. *Employment.* Many rehabilitation counselors provide a wide range of vocational and employment support services. Instructors can advise CITs to consider using TMH to deliver employment-related services. CITs should explore the pros and cons of TMH delivery depending on the type of vocational rehabilitation service provided (e.g., job search strategies, job development, job coaching).
7. *Transportation.* Part of independent living and working involves independent transportation. Many rehabilitation counselors assist clients with developing plans for transportation to home and work. Instructors can have CITs examine how they would support transportation planning when providing services via TMH, considering the pros and cons of delivering TMH services to address transportation planning.
8. *Housing.* Rehabilitation counselors may assist clients with developing plans for independent living. Instructors can have CITs examine how they would support independent living planning when providing services via TMH. CITs should address the pros and cons of delivering TMH services to support independent living planning.
9. *Collaborative Care.* Rehabilitation counseling often requires collaborative care between the counselor and service providers, such as housing specialists, mental health counselors, case managers, and medical providers. Instructors and CITs can explore how the use of TMH can be both a risk and a benefit to collaborative care models. Consider issues of access, security, and different TMH modalities.
10. *Continuum of Care.* Clinical rehabilitation is delivered in various settings, including primary care, outpatient, partial treatment, inpatient, integrated behavioral healthcare, and aftercare. Instructors and CITs can explore the risks and benefits of using TMH in different treatment settings. Consider issues of access, security, and different TMH modalities.

Sample Lesson: TMH Rehabilitation Counseling - Case Study, Questions, and Discussion

Heather C. Robertson, PhD, LMHC, CRC, NCC, BC-TMH
St. John's University

Lesson Objectives

At the end of this lesson, students will have

1) examined a case on delivering TMH Rehabilitation Counseling,
2) applied TMH concepts learned in the program to the case, and
3) decided on an ethical course of action regarding the case.

2024 CACREP Standards

Standards 5.G.5 (Rehabilitation counseling services and organizational settings, including independent living, community rehabilitation, and public/proprietary vocational rehabilitation programs), and 5.G.8 (Career- and work-related assessments, including job analysis, worksite modification, transferable skills analysis, job readiness, and work hardening).

Materials and/or Technology Required

Access to case study.

Preparation Required

Prior instruction on TMH and rehabilitation counseling.

Estimated Time Required for Lesson Delivery

Prior instruction time may vary. This activity should last approximately 30–45 minutes, depending on instructional time.

Structure and Audience for Lesson

This activity is best used in master's level Counselor training in Rehabilitation Counseling. Format can be in-person or online (synchronous or asynchronous).

Lesson Content and Instructional Strategies

Case Example

Quinn is a certified rehabilitation counselor (CRC) at a vocational rehabilitation organization. The organization has been providing telemental health (TMH) services since the COVID-19 pandemic. All staff are trained in TMH practice and are expected to adhere to the CRCC Code of Ethics (2023) Section K (Technology, Social Media, and Virtual Counseling). Quinn is working with Client D on vocational goals. Client D has a diagnosis of cerebral palsy, hearing loss for which they use hearing aids, and a wheelchair for mobility. Quinn and Client D have been working on job search strategies, interviewing skills, and self-advocacy for accommodations. Client D has a bachelor's degree in finance and is a recent college graduate. Client D received a job offer to work in a banking call center. The job allows for remote work, being issued a workplace laptop, and uses a proprietary software system. Client D is seeking support from Quinn on advocacy for workplace accommodations, including extended restroom breaks and the purchase of technology to enhance audio and visual capabilities for the software used. During the interview, the employer shared a link to a software demo, and Client D recognized that additional technology would be needed.

Quinn has been working with Client D via TMH since they began services. Client D would like to show Quinn the demo of the proprietary software to help them coordinate their self-advocacy. To access this demo, Client D has to sign on to a website where they must agree to maintain the privacy of the proprietary system. Client D stated they could share their screen with Quinn or email them their login/password for the demo so Quinn can get a sense of the system from the user end. Quinn states that it may be unethical or illegal for Client D to share the software and offers to connect with the employer on behalf of Client D to explain the need for the accommodation. Client D has not previously disclosed their disability to their employer and is uncomfortable with Quinn advocating on their behalf. Both Client D and Quinn feel that Quinn needs to see the software to be helpful in the self-advocacy process.

Questions

1. Assuming good intentions, what did Quinn do well?
2. What ethical issues were you aware of when reading the case? Consider both those that were adhered to and those that were possible risks.
3. What are your thoughts and feelings on using TMH with Client D based on their disability, functioning, and technological skills? What are the risks and benefits?
4. What are your thoughts and feelings on Client D sharing the proprietary software with Quinn? Are there any legal or ethical violations in Quinn's viewing of the software?
5. If you were Quinn, what other alternatives would you explore with Client D?

Discussion

1. Students review the case at the beginning of the lesson. The instructor may allow time for students to research the items in the case, such as Client D's disability.
2. Students can discuss the review questions above as a class, in pairs, or in small groups, and share their responses with the class. Online asynchronous classes may wish to use discussion boards to share their thoughts on the case.
3. The instructor can summarize the class's primary beliefs and place them into three categories: a) benefits, b) risks, and c) suggestions. This model allows students to recognize that TMH has both benefits and risks and to offer suggestions to Quinn.

Assessment of Objectives

Assessment of the lesson objectives can be conducted formally or informally. Informal assessment would involve group discussion via in-person or synchronous classes or online discussion boards for asynchronous classes. Instructors can adapt the assignment to a written paper, where students review the case and provide a summary of the discussion questions.

Sample Lesson: TMH Clinical Rehabilitation Counseling - Case Study, Questions, and Discussion

Heather C. Robertson, PhD, LMHC, CRC, NCC, BC-TMH
St. John's University

Lesson Objective(s)

At the end of this lesson, students will have

1) examined a case on delivering TMH rehabilitation counseling,
2) applied TMH concepts learned in the program to the case, and
3) decided on an ethical course of action regarding the case.

2024 CACREP Standards

Standards 5.D.4 (Rehabilitation service delivery systems, including housing, independent living, case management, public benefits programs, educational programs, and public/proprietary vocational rehabilitation programs); 5.D.5 (Clinical rehabilitation counseling services within the continuum of care, such as inpatient, outpatient, partial hospitalization and aftercare, integrated behavioral health care, and the rehabilitation counseling services networks).

Materials and/or Technology Required

Access to case study.

Preparation Required

Prior instruction on TMH and Clinical Rehabilitation Counseling.

Estimated Time Required for Lesson Delivery

Prior instruction time may vary. This activity should last approximately 30–45 minutes, depending on instructional time.

Structure and Audience for Lesson

This activity is best used in master's level counselor training in clinical rehabilitation counseling. Format can be in-person or online (synchronous or asynchronous).

Lesson Content and Instructional Strategies

Case Example

Quinn is a certified rehabilitation counselor (CRC) at a vocational rehabilitation organization. The organization has been providing telemental health (TMH) services since the COVID-19 pandemic. All staff are trained in TMH practice and are expected to adhere to the CRCC Code of Ethics (2023) Section K (Technology, Social Media, and Virtual Counseling). In Chapter 11, you met Client B, who has a diagnosis of Opioid Use Disorder, moderate, in early remission (*DSM-5,* F11.21), on maintenance therapy and medication-assisted treatment (MAT), specifically suboxone.

Client B is part of a veterans' drug treatment program due to their legal involvement and veteran status. Client B sustained a spinal cord injury/lumbar strain (L3 and L4 vertebrae injury) that resulted in medical discharge, surgery, and disability classification. Client B reports being prescribed opioids to treat back pain upon discharge, which eventually developed into addiction, including the misuse of prescription medication and the use of heroin/fentanyl.

Quinn received the information above via referral from Client B's addictions counselor, Taylor. Taylor is seeking collaborative treatment since a part of Client B's treatment plan involves vocational preparation. Client B is referred for a vocational intake, evaluation, workplace readiness, and job-seeking services. Quinn plans to deliver these services via TMH. Quinn informs Taylor that they can provide the vocational intake and evaluation for Client B via TMH and then assess which services would be appropriate for Client B based on the findings.

Questions

1. Assuming good intentions, what did Quinn do well?
2. What ethical issues were you aware of when reading the case? Consider both those that were adhered to and those that were possible risks.
3. What are your thoughts and feelings on using TMH with Client B based on their disability, functioning, and technological skills? What are the risks and benefits?
4. What other considerations are needed in this collaborative care model? Consider consent, disseminating reports, and TMH confidentiality and data security.
5. If you were Quinn, what concerns might you have about working with Client B? What strategies might you use for effective and ethical service provision?

Discussion

1. Students review the case at the beginning of the lesson. The instructor may allow students time to research the case items, such as Client B's disability, SUD, and MAT.
2. Students can discuss the review questions above as a class, in pairs, or in small groups, and share their responses with the class. Online asynchronous classes may wish to use discussion boards to share their thoughts on the case.
3. The instructor can summarize the class's primary beliefs and place them into three categories: a) benefits, b) risks, and c) suggestions. This model allows students to recognize that TMH has both benefits and risks and allows students to offer suggestions to Quinn.

Assessment of Objectives

Assessment of the lesson objectives can be conducted formally or informally. Informal assessment would involve group discussion via in-person or synchronous classes or online discussion boards for asynchronous classes. Instructors can adapt the assignment to a written paper, where students review the case and provide a summary of the discussion questions.

15

College and Student Affairs Counseling

Defining the scope of college counseling and student affairs is important before examining telemental health (TMH) practices. NASPA defines the role of the student affairs professional as "promoting student learning and development" (NASPA, n.d., para. 2) in higher education. CACREP's first standard within College Counseling and Student Affairs states that counselors-in-training (CITs) must learn "principles of student development and the effect on life, education, and career choices" (CACREP, 2023, p. 28). Student affairs and college counseling may include academic advising, career advising, student activities, student leadership development, residence life, Greek life, and other roles that support college student development. Despite its title of college counseling, student affairs and college counseling professionals may not necessarily be affiliated with college counseling offices, which typically require a mental health license to provide therapy unless the student affairs professional has a counseling license. They may work within college counseling centers, however, on programs such as sexual violence. I will continue to use the term TMH in this chapter with the understanding that distance work may not necessarily involve "mental health" counseling but other direct services, such as advising, student development, and mentorship. Regardless of the role, college student affairs counselors engage in TMH practice and must be trained to use ethical and effective distance services.

Key Concepts

CACREP Standards

CACREP Section 5.E (College Counseling and Student Affairs) outlines 10 learning outcomes in relation to College Counseling and Student Affairs. Like other sections of the standards, this specialization does not specifically address the use of TMH delivery. However, there are distinct and discernable connections to content on TMH in the College Counseling and Student Affairs Curriculum, as outlined in Table 15.1. If these concepts are unfamiliar, the instructor is encouraged to explore the training and reading materials suggested in Chapter 1.

Table 15.1

CACREP Section 5.E (College Counseling and Student Affairs) and Suggested TMH Content

CACREP Standards (2024)	Suggested TMH Content
5.E.1. Principles of student development and the effect on life, education, and career choices.	Applying TMH to various student development theories (e.g., Astin, 1984; Chickering & Reisser, 1993; Perry, 1968; Sanford, 1967; Tinto, 1987) and examining how each theory applies to distance delivery.
5.E.2. Organizational, management, and leadership theories relevant in higher education settings.	Administrative support for the provision of distance services; institutional information technology (IT) support for security and ethical standards; responding to needs of the student population; technological expectations of different college student populations; "digital immigrants/digital natives" (Prensky, 2001).

CACREP Standards (2024)	Suggested TMH Content
5.E.3. Organizational culture, budgeting and finance, and personnel practices in higher education.	Financial and IT support from the institution for providing distance services; willingness to invest in updated technology and software to reduce risk (Viano, 2023); risks of using personal devices for TMH practice.
5.E.4. Current trends in higher education.	Increasing trends toward online education and online students (Salama & Hinton, 2023); the necessity to provide support services to all students, including those online and those on-campus.
5.E.5. Diversity of higher education environments.	Awareness of student socioeconomic status and other demographic characteristics that may limit access to technology for the provision of distance services (see Chapter 4); racial identity models and the influence of TMH/distance delivery for diverse students (Sue, 2023).
5.E.6. The influence of institutional, systemic, interpersonal, and intrapersonal barriers on learning and career opportunities in higher education.	The ability of distance services and TMH to expand access to more services by eliminating geographic barriers, the possibility of connecting students to more diverse providers, cultural barriers to access (Sue, 2023).
5.E.7. Policies, programs, and services that are equitable, preventative, and responsive to the unique needs of students in higher education settings.	Safety and security precautions around student data and third-party vendors that support distance delivery of services (e.g., AlcoholEDU, Handshake; USED, 2023; Viano, 2023).
5.E.8. Higher education resources to improve student learning, personal growth, professional identity development, and mental health.	Benefits and risks of online distance services; e.g., benefits could include ease of access, reduced barriers, and risks could include data security, lack of engagement and personal connections.

CACREP Standards (2024)	Suggested TMH Content
5.E.9. Models of threat assessment and violence prevention in higher education settings.	Process of assessing for suicide/homicide in a distance/TMH format; contacting emergency resources for identified risk/threat from a distance (see safety planning in Chapter 13).
5.E.10. Roles of college counselors and student affairs professionals in collaborating with personnel from other educational settings to facilitate college and postsecondary transitions.	Capacity for TMH to increase collaboration among student affairs professionals and community partners; cautions regarding different ethical and professional standards among specializations (e.g., career counseling, advising, disability services); capacity for student affairs counselors to partner with other professionals via TMH, including career counselors (see Chapters 6 and 12) and school counselors (Chapter 17).

Distance Services for Online and On-Campus Students

The number of students enrolled in online education programs is growing. According to a 2019 (pre-COVID-19) *U.S. News and World Report* article, the 10 universities with the largest online enrollment ranged from 10,000 to 37,000 students (Moody, 2019). Compare those numbers to data from 2023, where one university enrolled over 65,000 students in its online programs (Arizona State University, 2023). Some argue that student affairs professionals are unprepared to meet online students' needs and are not being trained to address them (Stoller, 2019). Westra (2018) argues that any service available to on-campus students must be available to online students.

The COVID-19 pandemic required many universities to rapidly transition to online instruction. There is ample evidence to suggest that COVID-19 had a significant impact on the mental health of college students (Soira & Horgos, 2021) and specific populations, such as Black students (Jones et al., 2022), LGBTQ+ students (Gonzalez et al., 2023), and international students (Tozini & Castiello-Gutierrez, 2022). Paulino (2022) provides a variety of recommendations for student affairs professionals in the wake of COVID-19, suggesting that these practices are likely to impact future delivery. Some of these recommendations include 1) evaluating the platforms used to deliver distance services, 2) assessing technology options, 3) providing training on technology, 4) analyzing the effectiveness of support services online, and 5) creating online options for student engagement.

On-campus students also benefit from distance and TMH services. Access to virtual appointments and online interactive wellness programs can support on-campus students as well as online students. Many of Paulino's recommendations would apply when college counseling and student affairs services are provided virtually to on-campus students. In addition to ethical practice, college counselors and student affairs professionals must determine if services will be offered entirely online, only in person, or both. College counselors and student affairs professionals must establish equitable and fair policies for providing services across multiple formats. For instance, should online counseling be exclusive to online students or available to on-campus students as well?

Automated Distance Services

Many universities use third-party software to support the online services they provide to students, including various online automated services that improve access to resources for all students. These may include software products that support career services job postings, repositories for students to log service hours, scheduling systems, or portals for students to upload medical and disability records. Other products may include interactive educational programs on drug and alcohol use or sexual assault. While these technological tools may not be considered TMH or distance college counseling, they do support the remote provision of student affairs services to all students. Unfortunately, there have been instances of attacks by cyber criminals that could impact student data security (Viano, 2023). The U.S. Department of Education (USED) has developed requirements and guidelines for institutions receiving federal funding when contracting with third-party vendors (USED, 2023). As such, college counselors and student affairs professionals must consider the security of student data entered into these systems. Viano suggests strategies such as universities vetting third-party vendors and monitoring their data collection (2023). They must be aware of students' ability to reliably access the technology (see Chapters 4 & 14) needed for these services, particularly if they are mandatory.

Teaching Techniques

Instructors provide training on TMH and distance college counseling and student affairs services to CITs in various ways. Below is a list of suggested strategies that might reinforce instruction of TMH and distance practices for college counseling and student affairs. These strategies utilize andragogical principles, including self-motivated learning, using prior experiences, recognizing a need for information, and immediately applying learning in a real-world context (Knowles, 1975).

1. *Examining CAS Standards.* Instructors can advise students to review the Council for the Advancement of Standards (CAS, 2023) in Higher Education for their area of interest (e.g., advising, disability services, etc.). CITs should examine CAS standards for TMH and distance delivery content and/or consider how TMH and distance delivery could be used effectively within the suggested CAS standards for their functional area.
2. *Cultural Concepts.* CAS standards (https://www.cas.edu/standards.html) have been developed for various affinity groups, including students from diverse cultural and demographic identities, including disability, Indigenous, international, LGBTQ+, post-traditional, commuters, veteran and military, and women and gender programs. Instructors can advise CITs to examine the TMH literature to consider the effectiveness of distance practices with these diverse populations. CITs can discuss the pros and cons of distance student affairs services for each population.
3. *Automated Services and Third-Party Software.* CITs can identify 1–2 automated software products commonly used in higher education and examine the safety and security features provided by the vendor. This information may be identified on the vendor website and should include security features, the ability to obtain a business associate agreement (BAA), and any recent updates to the product.
4. *Examining Online Policies.* Instructors and CITs can explore posted policies at various institutions regarding access to online services. CITs can explore any policies posted within various institutions and offices regarding the use of online services for students.
5. *Debating Access to Online Services.* Instructors can advise CITs to engage in a debate about access to online services for on-campus students. CIT can be divided into small groups to research the pros and cons of providing online services to all students equally versus reserving online services for online students.
6. *Managing Crisis from a Distance.* One of the challenges of TMH and distance counseling is managing crises from a distance. Instructors and CITs can discuss the crises that may arise when

working with students online and how they would manage the crisis from a distance. Consider what precautions and policies could be used to mitigate risks.

7. *Student Engagement.* Providing distance college counseling and student affairs services may involve engaging students individually or in groups online. Instructors and CITs can discuss how to manage student disengagement from a distance, as well as strategies to increase students' engagement in online services.
8. *Americans with Disabilities Act (ADA) Accessibility.* TMH services must be provided using ADA-accessible software and resources. Instructors and CITs can evaluate the software tools used at their institution for alignment with ADA compliance (see resources in Chapter 14).
9. *Demographic Accessibility.* TMH services are only effective if the students have access to the technology needed to provide services. Instructors and CITs can examine the demographic makeup of students at their institution (typically posted through university institutional research) and discuss any potential barriers to TMH services based on the literature or technological infrastructure (see Chapter 4).
10. *Challenge and Support.* College counselors and student affairs professionals often use the challenge and support (Sanford, 1967) model in their work with college student development. Instructors and CITs can discuss how TMH and distance services can support college student development while also challenging them to transition into the world of work and independence. Discuss the pros and cons of delivering distance services as a supplement to both supporting and challenging students.

Sample Lesson: Assessing College Online Delivery Services

Joni O'Hagan, MSEd
St. John's University

Lesson Objective

After this assignment, students will have researched and reviewed online college services offered in college counseling and student affairs.

2024 CACREP Standards

Standard 5.E.4 (Awareness of current trends in higher education).

Materials and/or Technology Required

Online computer and internet access, and handout: ACPA Commission Areas.

Preparation Required

Students need prior instruction on providing distance services in the student affairs and college counseling environments.

Estimated Time Required

Students will spend approximately 1–2 hours researching college online services and engaging in an informational interview and 30 minutes sharing results (depending on class size).

Structure and Audience for Lesson

This activity best suits master's students enrolled in in-person or online graduate or professional development programs.

Lesson Content and Instructional Strategies

1. Context: Students would have previously received instruction on delivering college counseling and student affairs programs online. This lesson allows them to demonstrate learning by assessing college websites and online services.
2. Instructors assign students to work in pairs or small groups. If teaching online synchronously, students can utilize breakout rooms. If teaching asynchronously, the instructor can assign students/groups to work independently and share findings on a discussion board or another format.
3. Student groups/pairs will select two universities for the group/pair to evaluate. Ideally, each group/pair should examine different universities.
4. Using the ACPA Commission Areas handout, students should identify an area of college student services to evaluate an area of college student services to evaluate. Have each pair identify two universities and one functional area to evaluate. Each group should look at a different functional area and, ideally, other

institutions for as many areas as possible from the list (with the understanding that some universities may have different titles for these services).

5. Students will request, schedule, and conduct an informational interview to learn more about the area/university utilizing the virtual meeting platform offered if applicable. Specifically, for each area, pairs should consider asking or researching the questions at the bottom of the handout (see below).
6. At a follow-up class or later date, the instructor leads the class in a general discussion of the findings. While students cannot share all of the information they discovered, the instructor may want to ask: 1) Which functional area did they review, and how did they offer online services? 2) What patterns did you notice about the online services offered? 3) Name one strength and one concern you have about the online resources reviewed.

Assessment of Objective

Assessment of objective will be assessed via the student's classroom discussion/dialogue, or the results may be written and submitted for a grade.

Additional Resources

Handout: ACPA Commission Areas.

Handout: ACPA Commission Areas

https://myacpa.org/entities/commissions/

Academic Affairs

Academic Support

Admissions, Orientation, & 1st Year Experience

Assessment & Evaluation

Campus Safety

Career Services

Commuter Students

Counseling & Psychological Services

Faculty & Graduate Programs

Global Dimensions of Student Support

Graduate & Professional Student Affairs

Housing & Residence Life

Recreation, Athletics, & Wellness

Social Justice Education

Spirituality, Faith, Religion, & Meaning

Student Conduct

Student Involvement

1) Are any online services offered?
2) If yes, are they automated (e.g., no human interaction required)?
3) Are there any policies for accessing these services?
4) If virtual services are offered in-person, are there any posted policies on encryption or security of the software used?
5) Are any mobile apps (e.g., apps for wellness) or third-party software systems promoted (e.g., employer databases not owned by the school)?
6) If apps or third-party software are used, are there any policies posted on data collection, efficacy, or last updates?
7) Name one positive element among the tools you reviewed.
8) Name one caution or concern among the tools you reviewed.

Sample Lesson: Examining CAS Standards for Distance Guidance

Heather C. Robertson, PhD, LMHC, CRC, NCC, BC-TMH
St. John's University

Lesson Objective

After this assignment, students will have researched and reviewed Council for the Advancement of Standards in Higher Education (CAS, 2023) standards for guiding the provision of online student affairs services.

2024 CACREP Standards

Standard 5.E.8 (Higher education resources to improve student learning, personal growth, professional identity development, and mental health).

Materials and/or Technology Required

Access to CAS standards for various functional specializations, e.g., Disability Services, Fraternity and Sorority Life.

Preparation Required

Students need prior instruction on providing distance services in student affairs and college counseling environments.

Estimated Time Required

Varies depending on access to CAS standards and the nature of the assignment, e.g., in-class activity vs. take-home or assigned project.

Structure and Audience for Lesson

This activity best suits master's students enrolled in in-person or online college counseling and student affairs graduate programs.

Lesson Content and Instructional Strategies

1. Context: Students would have previously received instruction on delivering college counseling and student affairs programs online. They should also have had prior instruction on the Council for the Advancement of Standards in Higher Education standards (2023) for various functional areas of student affairs.

2. Instructors assign students to work in pairs, small groups, or individually. If teaching online synchronously, students can utilize breakout rooms. If teaching asynchronously, the instructor can assign students/groups to work independently and share findings on a discussion board or another format.
3. Students/groups/pairs will select one functional area to explore. If possible, the instructor should ensure that multiple functional areas are represented. A list of functional areas is available on the CAS website: https://www.cas.edu/standards.html
4. Students will review the CAS standards for their selected functional area. Specifically, students are reviewing the standards for discussion, guidance, and/or omission on the administration of these services online.

   Instructor Note: There is currently a fee to purchase CAS standards. However, students may access CAS standards in a variety of ways. Standards may be included in their textbooks or other learning materials. Additionally, students can communicate with student affairs professionals with access to CAS standards for their review.
5. Students should be considering the following questions during their review: a) What information is included on the online or distance delivery of services in the CAS standards, if any? b) How does the standard support TMH/distance services within this functional area? c) How would you implement TMH or distance standards within this domain while still supporting the CAS standards?
6. At a follow-up class/later date, the instructor leads the class in a general discussion of the findings. While students will not be able to share all the information they discovered, the instructor may want to ask: a) Which functional area did they review, and how did the standards address TMH? b) What concerns would you have about implementing TMH or online services within this domain while still adhering to the standards? c) Name one strength and one concern you have about the standards reviewed pertaining to TMH and distance delivery.

Assessment of Objective

The objective will be assessed via the student's classroom discussion/dialogue, or the results may be written and submitted for a grade.

16

Marriage, Couple, and Family Counseling

The concept of marriage, couples, and families has evolved. While not specific to telemental health (TMH) delivery, it is prudent to begin a discussion of marriage, couple, and family counseling by pointing out the potential barriers with the label of this specialization. Counselors-in-training (CITs) seeking to counsel individuals in relationships must recognize that *marriage* often assumes binary relationships such as "married" or "single." This term fails to include many clients who are cohabitating with a partner or partners with no goal, desire, or legal right to marry. The term *couple* implies a relationship with one other person when many people identify as polyamorous or polysexual (Barker & Iantaffi, 2019) and have meaningful romantic, emotional, or sexual relationships with several people. The term *family* can have different definitions, such as one's biological family versus one's chosen family. Even when clients have no identifiable biological family, they are raised within a system (e.g., family, foster system, ecosystem).

The terms *marriage, couple,* and *family* imply that biases exist within the field before the client even engages in counseling. Whether CITs provide services in-person or via TMH, the practice of marriage, couple, and family counseling is more inclusively defined as systems counseling or relational counseling. I use marriage, couple, and family (MC&F)

Counseling in this book for consistency and alignment with CACREP language. Yet, it is important to recognize the limits of these terms and consider altering terminology in our teaching and practice to create a more welcoming space for all. One of the benefits of TMH counseling is the capacity for clients to access more diverse providers with different skills, expertise, and professional training, as well as counselors with varied identities regarding relational or family systems. This includes counselors specializing in relational and systems counseling issues and those with welcoming and affirming practices.

Key Concepts

CACREP Standards

CACREP Section 5.F (Marriage, Couple, and Family Counseling) outlines 14 learning outcomes in relation to MC&F counseling. These standards do not specifically address the use of TMH delivery, yet they do address different service modalities, which may include TMH or face-to-face (F2F) modalities. In addition, there are distinct connections to TMH content in the MC&F curriculum, as outlined in Table 15.1. If these concepts are unfamiliar, the instructor is encouraged to explore the training and reading materials suggested in Chapter 1.

Table 15.1

CACREP 2024 Standards 5.F. (Marriage, Couple, and Family Counseling) and Suggested TMH Content

2024 CACREP Standards	Suggested TMH Content
5.F.1. Sociology of the family, family phenomenology, and family of origin theories.	Understanding technology in couple and family relationships (Herlein & Twist, 2019).
5.F.2. Aging and intergenerational influences and related family concerns.	Understanding aging and generational differences in the use of technology (Prensky, 2001), policies for working with minors and TMH, and determining appropriate TMH use based on the client's technological skills.

2024 CACREP Standards	Suggested TMH Content
5.F.3. Impact of interpersonal violence on marriages, couples, and families.	Challenges in assessing violence to self or others via TMH (see Chapter 9); capacity for TMH to increase access to support services (e.g., phone and text crisis lines); risk of creating digital footprint of internet searches (e.g., domestic violence support).
5.F.4. Interactions of career, life, and gender roles in marriages, couples, and families.	Recommend a review of Herlein and Twist (2019) *Chapter One, Couples, Family, and Technology*, including the prevalence of technology, mobile phones, video games, social networking, media, sedentary lifestyles, sleep, psychological well-being, life satisfaction, and work.
5.F.5. Impact of unemployment, under-employment, and changes in socioeconomic standing on marriages, couples, and families.	Understanding the digital divide (Chapter 4) and the limits to TMH MC&F counseling for groups from lower educational and socioeconomic backgrounds, as well as those lacking technological infrastructure; use of career development and career counseling TMH strategies (Chapters 6 and 12).
5.F.6. The impact of migration on family functioning.	Capacity for trauma to accompany migration and cautions for TMH use with trauma; adaptation of trauma treatments, e.g., eye movement desensitization and reprocessing (EMDR) therapy to TMH modalities; capacity for TMH to connect clients to multilingual providers.
5.F.7. Theories and models of marriage, couple, and family counseling.	Efficacy of TMH with MC&F counseling (McLean et al., 2021); exploring the application of TMH counseling to various MC&F theories; exploring the pros and cons of practicing theoretical approaches using different TMH modalities (e.g., phone, video, chat).

2024 CACREP Standards	Suggested TMH Content
5.F.8. Principles and models of assessment and case conceptualization from a systems perspective.	Adapting assessment and intake practices to TMH delivery with families (see Chapters 9, 13 & 14).
5.F.9. Family assessments, including genograms and family mapping.	Use of technology and TMH for family assessment, including collateral visits/engagement (IAMFC, 2017, Section E); tools for developing digital genograms.
5.F.10. Techniques and interventions of marriage, couple, and family counseling.	Adapting MC&F techniques to TMH delivery; adaptation of play therapy techniques (see lessons in this chapter).
5.F.11. Conceptualizing and implementing treatment, planning, and intervention strategies in marriage, couple, and family counseling.	Challenges when using TMH modalities (e.g., video, phone) for MC&F counseling stages; benefit of TMH to connect people to services, assessment, evaluation, and resources (e.g., psychiatrist, sex therapist).
5.F.12. Service delivery modalities and networks within the continuum of care, such as primary care, outpatient, partial treatment, inpatient, integrated behavioral healthcare, and aftercare.	"Service delivery models" include F2F and TMH treatment; TMH with different levels of care, e.g., providing TMH for outpatient care vs. using TMH for collateral or behavioral health integration for aftercare.
5.F.13. Strategies for interfacing with the legal system relevant to marriage, couple, and family counseling.	Encryption and security of transmitting and communicating court-ordered reports via secure technology; capacity for TMH to enhance collateral visits and family/child observations.
5.F.14. Third-party reimbursement and other practice and management issues in marriage, couple, and family counseling	Insurance, Medicaid, and Medicare definitions and reimbursement for TMH treatment; restrictions to reimbursement for TMH service delivery for MC&F counseling.

Establishment of TMH Guidelines in MC&F Counseling

Blumer et al. (2015) advocated for unified TMH MC&F training principles before COVID-19, and Hertlein et al. (2021) proposed that the need was more important than ever post-COVID. The American Association for Marriage and Family Therapy (AAMFT) Regulatory Boards (2016) established guidelines for teletherapy that included a wide range of practices. These practices included following the laws in each jurisdiction, counselor training, verifying client identity, client/counselor relationship, cultural competency, informed consent, limitations of TMH, confidentiality, boundaries, social media, sexual issues, documentation, billing, emergencies, synchronous and asynchronous services, the Health Insurance Portability and Accountability Act (HIPAA) security/encryption, archiving data, electronic links, testing and assessment, and tele-supervision. These guidelines reinforce practices and principles established by the International Association of Marriage and Family Counselors (IAMFC; 2017) and ACA (2014) Code of Ethics.

Challenges of TMH Play Therapy

One of the challenges of delivering family counseling via TMH is the use of play therapy. Play therapy techniques can be adapted to include online engagement and may even be enhanced using technological interventions. However, some play therapy elements, such as sand trays, dolls and manipulatives, or others, may be challenging to adapt to online delivery. Borenstein (2022) suggests adapting play with strategies such as allowing children to select the setting for their session (e.g., outside on a hammock, inside in a bedroom fort), allowing a child to share toys on screen, draw on screen, or use filters as toys. Smith et al. (2023) offer benefits and challenges to teleplay and contraindications. Some benefits include accessibility, viewing the family in their own home, and requiring parent engagement in session. Some challenges include having no physical interaction with the family, creating a safe environment in the family home, and hardware/software needs. Contraindications may include previous trauma or abuse inside the home, parents unwilling to engage in play, or determining whether in-person treatment is needed.

Teaching Techniques

Instructors can train MC&F CITs on TMH in a variety of ways. Below is a list of suggested strategies that might reinforce or supplement the instruction of TMH within the MC&F curriculum. These strategies utilize **andragogical** principles, including self-motivated learning, using prior experiences, recognizing a need for information, and immediately applying learning in a real-world context (Knowles, 1975).

1. *Examining Ethics.* MC&F counselors adhere to ethical guidelines published by ACA and the IAMFC but may also benefit from reviewing AAMFT codes. Instructors and CITs can review codes for guidance on TMH delivery, specifically IAMFC Section I: Technology Assisted Couples and Family Counseling (2017) and AAMFT Section VI, Technology-Assisted Professional Services (2015).
2. *Adapting Cases for TMH MC&F Counseling.* Instructors utilize case studies with CITs to demonstrate counseling scenarios. Instructors who use case studies can adapt their lessons such that CITs consider each case from both an F2F and TMH treatment lens, exploring the pros and cons of using TMH with each MC&F case.
3. *Setting the Stage for TMH Counseling.* MC&F counselors need to set the stage for clients at the first session, letting them know what they can expect during counseling. Instructors and CITs can explore how they would alter their opening remarks and guidelines for TMH sessions and explore how the opening discussion would vary for different modalities (e.g., phone, video, messaging).
4. *TMH Mock Family Sessions.* Instructors often use mock counseling sessions with CITs. CITs can practice providing mock family counseling sessions in various modalities, including video, phone, or chat, using the tools discussed in Chapter 2. The instructor can lead the class in a discussion of the strengths and weaknesses of their mock session, as well as opportunities to improve.
5. *TMH Mock Couple Sessions.* CIT can practice mock couples counseling sessions in various modalities, including video, phone, or chat, using the tools discussed in Chapter 2. The instructor can lead a discussion on the strengths and weaknesses of their mock session, as well as opportunities to improve.
6. *The Impact of Technology on the Family and/or Couple.* Hertlein and Twist (2019) recommend conducting an assessment of how technology impacts couple and family relationships and creating a technology plan with families and couples. Instructors can lead CITs in a discussion of how technology can impact families and couples. CITs can research evidence-based assessments that examine the impact of technology on couples and families. CITs can practice developing technology plans with families, including both F2F and TMH practice sessions.

7. *Couples/Relationships and Technology.* Some couples or relational conflicts may involve technology. Examples include online infidelity, sexting, monitoring and tracking partners via phone, or the viewing of online pornography. In TMH, the conduit for these conflicts (e.g., phone, computer) also serves as access to treatment. Instructors and CITs can explore the risks and benefits of using TMH in couples/relational counseling when the source of the conflict stems from the use of technology.
8. *Evaluating Online Genogram Tools.* A genogram is a standard family assessment tool that helps the counselor and client understand family dynamics and relationships. Various tools exist that create online genograms. CITs can select one online genogram tool and evaluate it for its effectiveness, security, and ease of use in both F2F and TMH counseling sessions. CITs can conduct mock TMH sessions with peers using genogram software to fully evaluate its utility in practice.
9. *Translating Family Theories to TMH.* Instructors provide content to CITs on various types of family therapy, including Bowenian, Structural, Systemic, and others. CITs can examine the efficacy of using TMH with each theoretical modality and consider the challenges and strengths of adapting the approach to TMH delivery.
10. *Deciding to Deliver TMH MC&F Counseling.* Families and couples are composed of diverse individuals with different needs, abilities, strengths, and levels of functioning. The MC&F counselor is charged with determining if TMH is an appropriate modality for the client(s). Instructors and CITs can discuss various elements that support and or discourage the use of TMH with couples and families. Consider elements such as age, ability, geographic location, access to technology, and the need for all members to access technology equally.

Sample Lesson: Adapting Play Therapy Techniques to TMH

Michelle Perepiczka, PhD, LMHC, LPC, RPT-S, ACS, NCC
University of Phoenix

Lesson Objective

At the end of this lesson, students will have explored strategies for adapting in-person play therapy techniques to distance delivery via TMH.

2024 CACREP Standards

Standard 5.F.10 (Techniques and interventions of marriage, couple, and family counseling).

Materials and/or Technology Required

Online computer and internet access.

Preparation Required

Students need prior instruction on providing marriage, couple, and family ounseling via TMH and some of the unique elements of delivery play therapy online.

Estimated Time Required for Lesson Delivery

Students engage in a 15–30 minute research and creativity session, as well as a 15–30 minute sharing discussion.

Structure and Audience for Lesson

This activity is best suited for master's students enrolled in in-person or online graduate programs or professional development programs.

Lesson Content and Instructional Strategies

1. Context: Students have received earlier instruction on the pros, cons, and ethics of distance marriage, couple, and family counseling, as well as the unique elements of adapting play therapy to online delivery.
2. Students will work in pairs or small groups (self-selected or assigned by the instructor).
3. Students will select one play therapy technique or intervention (self-selected or assigned by the instructor) primarily delivered in person but may be adapted to online delivery. Ideally, a variety of techniques should be selected to avoid repetition.
4. In groups or pairs, students will research and brainstorm strategies to adapt the in-person play therapy technique to online delivery. Students will need to address:
    a. Name of play therapy technique selected and its clinical purpose.

   b. What cautions, ethics, and safety protocols should the counselor consider when adapting this technique to online instruction?
   c. How would the counselor adapt this technique to TMH? Consider different delivery modalities, including synchronous online video or phone sessions, and determine if the technique could be delivered asynchronously.
   d. What technology and tools do the counselor need to adapt the technique? What technology and tools do they need the client to have?
   e. Be prepared to model the online adaptation with the class.
5. When the pairs/groups have spent sufficient time reviewing and brainstorming their play therapy techniques, the larger class resumes, and the instructor leads a discussion based on the following:
   a. What ethical issues did you encounter in attempting to adapt your intervention?
   b. Was your adaptation effective? Which modality was most effective?
   c. How would you feel about using this adapted intervention with clients?
   d. How would you feel if a counselor used this adapted intervention with you as the client or with a family member?
   e. Name one pro and one con of adapting the intervention to an online delivery modality.

Assessment of Objectives

The objective will be assessed via the students' classroom discussion/dialogue, or their adaptations may be written down or modeled and video-recorded in a presentation format to be submitted for a grade.

Sample Lesson: Mini-Practice in Applying Play Therapy Techniques Adapted to TMH

Michelle Perepiczka, PhD, LMHC, LPC, RPT-S, ACS, NCC, University of Phoenix
Kami Ball Tran, MS, LPC-S, RPT-S, NCC

Lesson Objective

At the end of this lesson, students will have practiced implementing strategies for adapting in-person play therapy techniques to distance delivery via TMH.

2024 CACREP Standards

Standard 5.F.10 (Techniques and interventions of marriage, couple, and family counseling).

Materials or Technology Required

Online computer and internet access, as well as basic play therapy materials, such as art supplies, toys, or symbolic items, to create a therapeutic environment.

Preparation Required

Students need prior instruction on providing marriage, couple, and family counseling via TMH, play therapy basic skills, and some of the unique elements of delivering play therapy online.

Estimated Time Required for Lesson Delivery

Students engage in a 15–20 minute mock play therapy session, as well as a 15–30 minute sharing discussion.

Structure and Audience for Lesson

This activity is best suited for master's students enrolled in in-person or online graduate programs or professional development programs.

Lesson Content and Instructional Strategies

1. Context: Students have earlier received instruction on play therapy basic skills and theory, the ethics of distance marriage,

couple, and family counseling, and the unique elements of adapting play therapy to online delivery.

2. Students will work in partners (self-selected or assigned by the instructor).
3. Students will select one play therapy technique or intervention (self-selected or assigned by the instructor) and practice implementing it via TMH.
4. Students will record their mock sessions to receive feedback from their peers and supervision from their instructor.
5. Students in the client role will set up their designated play therapy space and ensure that all necessary materials are within reach for the person in the mock client role. The mock client's camera will be positioned so the mock therapist is able to see the full space with the therapeutic toys.
6. When the pairs have spent sufficient in their mock role plays and have each taken a turn in the play therapist role, the larger class resumes, and the instructor leads a discussion based on the following:
    a. What play therapy intervention was selected to be implemented via TMH? What was the rationale for the choice?
    b. What challenges did you face in preparing and setting up the play therapy space at home, and how did it impact the overall session?
    c. Reflect on the use of play therapy materials during the online session. How did the virtual environment affect how the client utilized these materials, and what adjustments did you make?
    d. In what ways did the choice of play therapy skills utilized contribute to building rapport and engagement with your practice partner during the online play therapy session?
    e. Consider the technological aspect of the session. Were there any unexpected issues with connectivity or the technology, and how did you address them to ensure a smooth session?
    f. Reflect on the importance of ethical considerations in TMH play therapy, particularly concerning using play therapy materials. How did you navigate issues related to confidentiality and ethical guidelines during the session?

Assessment of Objective

The objective will be assessed via the students' classroom discussion/dialogue and/or their video-recorded session to be submitted for a grade.

17

School Counseling

Professional school counselors are licensed or certified school professionals who assist students in attaining academic, career, and personal/social goals. According to the American School Counselor Association (ASCA), school counselors "design and deliver school counseling programs that improve student outcomes" (ASCA, 2023, p. 2). Before the pandemic, school counselors were engaged in telemental health (TMH) and distance counseling, specifically for those working with homeschooled students, students in medical settings, and students in remote or online schools. Counselors-in-training (CITs) who pursue a career as professional school counselors must understand the nuances of distance school counseling as they seek to engage students in all settings. In this chapter, I intentionally use the terms "distance counseling" or "distance delivery" instead of telemental health (TMH) counseling. While school counselors have an active role in helping students maintain emotional wellness and screening those with mental health conditions, treatment for mental health conditions is often relegated to other professionals within the school (e.g., social worker, psychologist) or referred to out-of-school providers.

Key Concepts

CACREP Standards

CACREP Standards Section 5.H (School Counseling) outlines 19 learning outcomes in relation to School Counseling curricula. These standards do not specifically address the use of distance or digital counseling; however, there are opportunities for instructors to connect content on TMH into the school counseling curriculum, as outlined in Table 17.1. If suggested concepts are unfamiliar, the instructor is encouraged to explore the training and reading materials suggested in Chapter 1. Many of the CACREP standards closely align with the American School Counselor Association (ASCA) Ethical Standards, specifically A.15 (Technical and Digital Citizenship) and A.16 (Virtual/Distance School Counseling) (ASCA, 2022). Since school counselor education programs provide instruction on ASCA ethics, references to ASCA codes are included in relation to the CACREP standards below.

Table 17.1

CACREP Section 5.C, Clinical Mental Health Counseling (CMHC) and Suggested TMH Content

CACREP Standards (2024)	Suggested TMH Related Content
5.C.1. Models of school counseling programs.	Developing effective distance school counseling programs that "Adhere to the same legal and ethical standards in a virtual/distance/hybrid setting as in face-to-face settings" (ASCA, A.16.a).
5.C.2. Models of PK–12 comprehensive career development.	Considering the appropriateness of distance school counseling at various grade levels based on access and ability; distance Career Counseling (see Chapters 6 and 12).
5.C.3. Models of school-based collaboration and consultation.	Capacity for distance school counseling services to increase collaboration and consultation while also considering risks. "Recognize, acknowledge and problem-solve the unique challenges and limitations of virtual/distance/hybrid school counseling" (ASCA, A.16.b).

CACREP Standards (2024)	Suggested TMH Related Content
5.C.4. Development of school counseling program mission statements and objectives.	Determining if distance school counseling services would support the mission and objectives of the school, the counseling office, students, parents, and the surrounding community.
5.C.5. Design and evaluation of school counseling curriculum, lesson plan development, diverse classroom management strategies, and differentiated instructional strategies.	Considering all safety precautions in developing distance school counseling programs, including challenges and limitations (ASCA, A.16.A.b), confidentiality, and unintended viewers or recipients (ASCA, A.16.d).
5.C.6. School counselor roles as leaders, advocates, and systems change agents in PK–12 schools.	Utilizing distance counseling as a change agent to support students and families, and access community collaborators.
5.C.7. Qualities and styles of effective leadership in schools.	Connection between self-care and effective leadership; capacity for distance counseling to blur work/life boundaries. School counselor self-care and distance counseling (Kus & Aydin, 2022; Villares et al., 2022). "Advocate against alert tools or apps requiring constant monitoring by school personnel. These tools are not aligned with the nature and function of school counseling" (ASCA, A.15.i).
5.C.8. Advocacy for comprehensive school counseling programs and associated school counselor roles.	"Advocate for equitable access to technology for all students" (ASCA, A.15.a).
5.C.9. School counselor roles and responsibilities in relation to the school crisis and management plans.	Challenges in facilitating crisis management via virtual services (see ASCA, A.16.g.); "Establish procedures, in collaboration with school administrators and other support staff, for students to follow in both emergency and non-emergency situations when the school counselor is not available" (ASCA, A16.c).

CACREP Standards (2024)	Suggested TMH Related Content
5.C.10. School counselor consultation with families, PK–12 and postsecondary school personnel, community agencies, and other referral sources.	Capacity for distance counseling to support consultation; "inform both students and parents/guardians of the benefits and limitations of virtual/distance/hybrid school counseling" (ASCA, A.16.e.)
5.C.11. Skills to critically examine the connections of social, cultural, familial, emotional, and behavioral factors to academic achievement.	"Demonstrate appropriate selection and equitable use of culturally sustaining technology and software applications to enhance students' academic, career and social/emotional development" (ASCA, A.15.b).
5.C.12. Skills to screen PK–12 students for characteristics, risk factors, and warning signs of mental health and behavioral disorders.	Challenges in facilitating crisis management via virtual services (see ASCA, A.16.g, "Recognize the challenges in virtual/distance/hybrid settings of assisting students considering suicide…").
5.C.13. Strategies for implementing and coordinating school-based interventions.	"Educate students on how to participate in the electronic school counseling relationship to minimize and prevent potential misunderstandings that could occur due to lack of verbal cues and inability to read body language or other visual cues that provide contextual meaning to the school counseling process and relationship" (ASCA.A.16.f).
5.C.14. Techniques of social-emotional and trauma-informed counseling in school settings.	Challenges within distance counseling to recognize verbal cues that indicate trauma and/or distress (see ASCA, A.16.f).
5.C.15. Evidence-based and culturally sustaining interventions to promote academic development.	"Demonstrate appropriate selection and equitable use of culturally sustaining technology and software applications to enhance students' academic, career and social/emotional development" (ASCA, A.15.b).

CACREP Standards (2024)	Suggested TMH Related Content
5.C.16. Approaches to increase promotion and graduation rates.	Capacity for technology (not specifically distance counseling) to support academics (e.g., online tutoring tools); school counselors' ability to share these resources with students to support their academic growth.
5.C.17. Interventions to promote postsecondary and career readiness.	Myriad ways in which career counseling and college search processes are facilitated by technology and distance counseling; school counselors' ability to share and train students on these resources (see Chapters 6 and 12).
5.C.18. Strategies to facilitate school and postsecondary transitions.	Capacity for technology (not specifically distance counseling) to support college and job searchers (e.g., online information); school counselors' ability to share these resources with students during distance services to support transitions.
5.C.19. Strategies to promote equity in student achievement and access to postsecondary education opportunities.	Capacity for distance counseling to promote equal access to counseling services and parental conferences if technology is accessible.

School Policy

It is prudent that schools create distance counseling school policies outlining the conditions under which distance counseling will be utilized and the parameters guiding its use. These policies should be informed by the ASCA Code of Ethics, Sections A.15 (Digital Citizenship) and A.16. (Virtual/Distance School Counseling). Policies should specify under which conditions distance school counseling will be utilized. For example, will distance school counseling be a regular offering for all students, including those physically located in the school? Will it be used for parental and third-party consultations? Is it only used in a crisis, home-schooling, or for students who are home due to medical needs? If so, how would "crisis" be defined? Schools should seek legal counsel on any policies involving distance services, particularly regarding the privacy of student information. School policies should specify what types of information may or may not be shared with school counselors. While distance counseling creates convenience for parents and students to access school counselors, it may present boundary issues for school counselors and impact counselor burnout.

School Counselor Wellness

Let's examine the impact of distance services on school counselor wellness. Since COVID-19, several studies have examined the impact of distance counseling in school settings and its effect on counselor wellness. One caveat is that these studies were conducted either during or immediately following the national COVID crisis. During this time, it is likely that all professionals—school counselors and otherwise—were experiencing stress. Nonetheless, the findings of these studies are important for CITs considering engaging in distance school counseling. Studies have shown that school counselors utilize the same counseling skills during distance school counseling as they do during in-person counseling, with some studies indicating a greater need for flexibility and follow-up during distance services (Abdallah Altarawneh & Awwad Alomoush, 2022; Al-Halalmeh & Al-Halalmeh, 2021).

School counselor burnout was examined in relation to providing distance services. Some studies suggest that school students were unmotivated participants compared to other clients in distance counseling services (Barker & Barker, 2022). Other studies focused on the challenge of distance delivery, including work-life balance, learning virtual technology, legal concerns, and using counseling skills in a virtual setting (Hornor & Westberry, 2023). In another study, the size of the school counselor caseload and their prior training in trauma was found to be insignificant in school counselors' delivery of digital services, yet taking time away from school counseling duties to engage in administrative services impacted school counselor effectiveness (Villares et al., 2022). Other research cited digital fatigue as impacting digital school counselor wellness (Kus & Aydin, 2022). These studies emphasize that, like all counseling practices, digital delivery of school counseling requires attention to overall counselor wellness.

Teaching Techniques

School CITs can receive instruction on distance school counseling in various ways. Below is a list of suggested strategies that might reinforce or supplement the instruction of distance counseling in school counseling curricula. These strategies utilize andragogical principles, including self-motivated learning, using prior experiences, recognizing a need for information, and immediately applying learning in a real-world context (Knowles, 1975).

1. *Examining Ethics.* As always, it is recommended that instructors teach ASCA Ethical Codes, with particular emphasis on A.15 and A.16. Table 17.1 provides suggestions on how the ASCA ethical codes can be integrated with CACREP standards and information on distance/virtual counseling. Yet CITs and instructors can examine these codes in relation to others (e.g., ACA, 2014) or current practices in their school/internship.
2. *Academic.* A primary function of the school counselor is to support students in their academic progress. Instructors can facilitate discussion on how distance counseling can support students with academic struggles, including risks and benefits. CITs can role-play mock distance counseling sessions focused on academic concerns.
3. *Career.* School counselors support students in their career and post-secondary planning. Instructors can facilitate discussion on how distance counseling can support students with career and post-secondary planning issues, including risks and benefits. CITs can role-play mock distance counseling sessions focused on career concerns, using tools and strategies discussed in Chapters 6 and 12.
4. *Social/Emotional.* School counselors support students with social/emotional concerns. Instructors can facilitate discussion on how distance counseling can support students with social/emotional concerns, including risks and benefits, as well as maintaining their scope of practice within school policies. CITs can role-play mock distance counseling sessions focusing on social/emotional concerns.
5. *Consent and Assent.* Instructors can advise CITs to consider how parental consent and student assent issues would vary when providing virtual services as opposed to in-person services. CIT can explore what information would be added to consent documents and how and where that information would be shared with parents and students.
6. *Parental Meetings.* Instructors and CITs can explore the pros and cons of using virtual counseling services for meetings with parents and guardians. What is gained or lost by meeting with

parents and guardians virtually instead of their coming to school? How does parental access to technology impact these practices?

7. *Classroom Guidance.* School counselors are responsible for delivering classroom guidance lessons. Instructors regularly require CITs to develop guidance lessons as a part of their training. Instructors can add an element to those assignments by having CITs adapt their guidance lesson for online delivery to either students or parents.
8. *Assessing Student Outcomes.* The ASCA National Model emphasizes student outcomes and the school counselor's role in assessing student outcomes. Instructors and CITs can explore ways distance school counseling creates data for evaluating student outcomes. Consider both the risks and benefits of using distance school counseling to collect data for assessment purposes.
9. *College and Career Search.* Some schools utilize college counselors and professional school counselors to support post-secondary transitions. Instructors can facilitate discussion on how distance counseling can support students' college search and application process, considering the multitude of resources available online. Other scenarios could involve students preparing to enter the workforce post-high school. CITs can role-play mock distance counseling sessions focused on post-secondary planning.
10. *Data Security Audit.* Many schools use third-party software tools to support their school counseling programs, including both in-person and virtual services. These may include email, cloud storage, video conferencing, college or employment search databases, grade portals, or other software tools. Instructors can advise CITs to identify as many third-party software products as possible at their field placement site (or from the school where they were students). CITs can conduct a mock software audit, seeking information on data security and encryption features such as Family Educational Rights and Privacy Act (FERPA) and Health Insurance Portability and Accountability Act (HIPAA) compliance.

Sample Lesson: Tech Awareness & Decision Making

Cameka Hazel, EdD, MHC-LP, New York Institute of Technology
Claudette Brown-Smythe, PhD, LMHC, ACS, NCC, CRC, SUNY Brockport

Lesson Objectives

1) Students will explain the importance of utilizing security and privacy feature settings for the safe delivery of telehealth.
2) Students will discuss ASCA ethical standards regarding school counselors' role when using digital technology.
3) Students will generate strategies to promote positive social interaction on social media.

2024 CACREP Standards

None.

ASCA Ethical Standards (2022)

Standards A.15 (Technical and Digital Citizenship) and A.16 (Virtual/Distance School Counseling).

Materials and/or Technology Required

ASCA Ethical Standards (2022), and the FERPA and HIPAA compliance policies.

Preparation Required

This lesson requires knowledge of ethical codes related to the digital delivery of school counseling. Specifically, knowledge of ASCA Ethical Standards A.15 (Technical and Digital Citizenship) and A.16 (Virtual/Distance School Counseling); knowledge and understanding of **FERPA** and HIPAA compliance policies.

Estimated Time Required for Lesson Delivery

Approximately 2 hours.

Structure and Audience for Lesson

This lesson is structured to be delivered in all formats for counselors in training.

Lesson Content

1. Utilizing security and privacy features settings for safe delivery of telehealth services.
    - Observe the age requirement for social media sites and apps.

- Use password-encrypted software and apps. Encryptions keep data safe and inaccessible from others on the internet.
- Per HIPAA regulations, schools should avoid storing data on personal devices, especially when shared with others. Institutions should provide a host or cloud to store information.
- Do not leave students' information open and accessible on devices; only use secure websites with a lock icon in the address bar.
- Ensure devices are updated with new programs and antivirus software to increase safety.
- Use passwords for wireless connections and avoid using public Wi-Fi to access telehealth services.

2. Understand ethical standards regarding the school counselor's role when using digital technology (ASCA Ethical Standards A.15 and A.16, FERPA, and HIPAA).
    - Adhere to school and district-wide policies for online service/activities delivery. School counselors need to be familiar with the platforms and knowledgeable of the privacy policies and limitations of the platform used by the school. As per FERPA regulations, the school counselor should advocate for changes if the platform violates the integrity of students' records and privacy.
    - Parents sign and release informed consent so the student can engage in telehealth.
    - Educate students regarding boundary setting in a virtual environment.
    - Place information regarding telehealth on the schools' websites and consistently update them.
    - Check in with clients about their current location. This will help in case of an emergency.
    - Discuss limits to confidentiality when providing online services/activities with students and plans on how to mitigate these limits.
    - School counselors should use private spaces and devices that increase privacy and confidentiality if not in a private location.

- School counselors should ensure professional boundaries and professional distance from students and parents (as per ASCA Standard A.5).

3. Apply strategies to promote positive social interaction on social media.
   - Creativity for the clinician is very important. Engaging children in a virtual environment can be more challenging than in person. Children can face boredom and feel distant. School counselors can use role play, virtual board games, virtual stories and songs, digital interactive notebooks, prerecorded guided imagery, and relaxation activities to keep students engaged.
   - School counselors should establish rules for effective communication and engagement in sessions, e.g., keeping the camera on, dress attire, waiting on one's turn to speak, keeping the background uncluttered and noise-free, and being transparent about who else is hearing the student's conversation in their background.

Instructional Strategies

Case Example

Alix is a 16-year-old high school student at Amity High. He was recently transitioned into the school's online program due to high levels of social anxiety. He has been receiving counseling from his school counselor for the past two years. He shared with her that he has suffered rejection from his parents, verbal abuse, has suicide ideations, and smokes marijuana daily.

Mrs. Hickory, Alix's school counselor, had just finished a telecounseling session with him. She was in her office at Amity High, while Alix attended the session virtually from home. After the session, Mrs. Hickory received a call from the principal to participate in a brief meeting. She left the office without securing her computer. On returning to her office, Michael came to her for assistance in completing his college board application, due that day. Michael did not have access to a computer and asked Mrs.

Hickory for permission to quickly use her computer to submit his college application. Upon receiving permission, Michael jumped on her computer and proceeded to the college board website. Mrs. Hickory was then paged to go to the principal's office and left Michael in the office on the computer. Michael became curious and started looking at the files and web pages Mrs. Hickory had open. He came upon her notes regarding Alix's session. When Mrs. Hickory returned, Michael began to talk about Alix and shared that he did not know his friend was going through so much. It was during this conversation that he revealed that he had read the notes she had on the computer about Alix. Suddenly, Mrs. Hickory realized she had not secured the student information and her files before leaving the room.

Step 1. The instructor will provide students with a copy of the case example to review. After reviewing the case, the instructor will discuss key concepts regarding security and privacy features in telehealth and the school counselor's role when using digital technology.

Step 2. Complete group assignment on security and privacy and ASCA, HIPAA, and FERPA standards. Students will work in groups to discuss the following questions. Instructors should encourage students to identify a recorder and a presenter. Students will need access to ASCA Ethical Standards (2022), the FERPA privacy act, and the HIPAA compliance policy for digital delivery.

Questions

1. What privacy and safety features should Mrs. Hickory have used to safeguard her work computer and student information, e.g., ASCA A.15.c?
2. Identify at least five ASCA ethical standards regarding the school counselor's role when using digital technology.
3. Discuss how Mrs. Hickory and Michael violated HIPAA and FERPA policies.

Step 3. Review and discussion of group assignment. The instructor will have students share their answers with the whole group and follow up on questions and/or observations posed by students.

Step 4. Discussion on strategies to promote positive social interaction on social media. The instructor will facilitate a large group discussion utilizing questions to reinforce concepts related to digital delivery, e.g., anonymity, confidentiality, boundary setting in **social media**, or password-protected devices. Sample questions: thinking about your usage of social media, e.g., Facebook, Twitter, Instagram, LinkedIn, Snapchat, TikTok:

1. What practices do users engage in on social media that could impact the effectiveness of your work with clients?
2. What are creative ways to ensure effective communication when working with students online in group counseling or individual counseling?
3. What are some ground rules you can establish between you and the client?

Assessment of Objectives

Students will be assessed on the objectives based on the discussion questions and their ability to identify and apply relevant ASCA ethical standards and related policies and generate strategies to promote positive social interaction on social media.

References

The "School Counselor and Virtual School Counseling" position statement (ASCA, 2017) https://www.schoolcounselor.org/Standards-Positions/Position-Statements/ASCA-Position-Statements/The-School-Counselor-and-Virtual-School-Counseling.

Sample Lesson: Facilitating Online Classroom Guidance Lessons

Gina Cicco, EdD, LMHC, NCC, Certified School Counselor
St. John's University

Lesson Objectives

1) Students will be able to identify the hallmarks of effective online instructional models needed to deliver online classroom guidance lessons;

2) students will be able to discuss the importance of rapport-building in online supervisory relationships; and
3) students will be able to provide examples effective communication and leadership patterns in online courses, such as the PICCA (Presence, Interaction, Clarity, Consistency, and Availability) Model.

2024 CACREP Standards

Standards 3.A.12 (The purpose of and roles within counseling supervision in the profession) and 5.H.7 (Qualities and styles of effective leadership in schools).

Materials and/or Technology Required

Zoom, Microsoft Teams, or WebEx; PowerPoint; learning management system (LMS), e.g., Canvas, Blackboard.

Preparation Required

Students will be assigned to read the following articles in preparation for the lesson and asked to adapt the content review from a college classroom to a school counselor guidance lesson:

Cicco, G. (2019). Effective communication in online courses: A self-assessment guide for instructors. *i-manager's Journal of Educational Technology, 20*(3), 1–6.

Cicco, G. (2017). Establishing positive culture and climate in the online classroom: Pathways for instructors. *i-manager's Journal of Educational Technology, 14*(2), 1–5.

The above reading assignments and corresponding review questions will be posted on the LMS course shell at the start of the course or at least two weeks in advance of the synchronous lesson. Students will reflect on its application to school classroom guidance lessons.

Estimated Time Required for Lesson Delivery

Two hours.

Structure and Audience for Lesson

Synchronous online setting, graduate students.

Lesson Content and Instructional Strategies

PowerPoint, small-group exercises.

1. The instructor will discuss various effective online instructional strategies, including data models to support these best practices.
2. Effective communication and leadership techniques for use within online classroom guidance will be reviewed, such as incorporating structure and roadmaps, offering opportunities for regular feedback, dyadic and triadic student/counselor interactions, posting regular reminders and updates, and integrating varied media to accommodate student learning styles and preferences, as needed during online classroom guidance lessons.
3. The PICCA Model will be reviewed in a PowerPoint presentation to highlight the importance of instructor presence, interaction, clarity, consistency, and availability in online classroom guidance lessons.
4. Online classroom climate and culture will be explained and discussed as fundamental to student learning outcomes, utilizing the articles assigned as supplemental readings in preparation for the lesson as resources.
5. The purpose and evolution of school counselor trustworthiness, competence, authenticity, and purposeful rapport-building practices will be emphasized as necessary and essential for counselor growth and development.
6. Effective supervision, leadership, and instructional practices will be discussed in the context of small working groups via breakout rooms.
7. During the small-group exercise, students will be encouraged to share ideas about how to apply these skills in real-life school counseling roles and practice delivery of classroom guidance lessons.

Assessment of Objectives

- Comprehension questions will be generated throughout the lesson.
- During breakout rooms, each small group will be presented with a brief case study that depicts school counselor/student interaction in an online course setting and will then critique the school counselor's response to student concerns posed in the case study.

- Students' responses during the breakout room activity will be indicative of their comprehension of the lecture and discussion sections of the lesson on online guidance lesson, rapport-building, communication, and leadership skills.
- Students in each breakout room will have designated roles as the group reporter and recorder and will then share a brief summary of their group's work with the larger group as a whole. Journaling and creativity of small-group summaries will be encouraged.

Other Considerations

18

Professional Practice and Fieldwork

All counseling master's programs, regardless of specialization, require counselors-in-training (CITs) to practice counseling skills in real-world settings. This real-world practice may be called practicums, internships, fieldwork, or other terms. Master's programs accredited by CACREP require that students engage in three fieldwork experiences, including one practicum and two internships. CACREP outlines these clinical experiences in Standard 4, Professional Practice (2024). As telemental health (TMH) practice continues to expand following the COVID-19 pandemic (Alvarado, 2021; American Psychiatric Association, 2021), CITs continue to engage in TMH practice during their fieldwork experiences. In addition, site and faculty supervisors engage in virtual/distance supervision, often termed *e-supervision* or *tele-supervision*. While e-supervision is discussed in Chapter 19, a full review of e-supervision practices is beyond the scope of this book.

Monitoring the professional practice of CITs involves more than teaching students during a fieldwork seminar class. Counselor education programs spend significant time, energy, and preparation establishing field placement standards and procedures for students and community supervisors. These field placement experiences may be managed by specific faculty member(s) or the field placement coordinator. The infusion of TMH into professional practice happens long before students enter their fieldwork seminar class and continues beyond the seminar hours. Sections 2 and 3 of this book outline how TMH should be a component of both the generalized and specialized counseling curriculum. The infusion of TMH into professional practice is an integral part of program planning and policy development, much like the fieldwork experiences themselves.

CACREP Curricular Standards

The CACREP standards outlined in Section 4 are not strictly learning objectives and content for instruction but involve organizing and administering the fieldwork experiences. Throughout this book, I focused primarily on teaching TMH concepts in the classroom. However, in this chapter, I address how TMH can and should be infused into the professional practice component of counselor education programs. Instead of providing a table of TMH recommendations aligned with the CACREP standards, I will discuss how TMH elements can be embedded into the program administration, fieldwork seminar instruction, and communication with supervisors.

Program Administration

Support for field placement. CACREP Standard 4.A states, "The counselor education program provides ongoing support to help students find fieldwork sites that are to provide the quality, quantity, and variety of expected experiences to prepare students for their roles and responsibilities as professional counselors..." (2024). Counselor education programs tracking fieldwork sites should determine if ethical TMH services are offered at these sites. While CACREP does not require TMH services, this standard suggests that programs prepare CITs for various roles and responsibilities, including TMH. Similarly, counselor education programs may need to establish policies on field placement sites that provide only TMH and determine if those sites adequately prepare CITs for various roles and responsibilities. This information is communicated to CITs as they begin their field placement experiences.

Insurance. Standard 4.B specifies, "Students are covered by individual professional counseling liability insurance while enrolled in practicum and internship." Counselor education programs are responsible for ensuring that student malpractice insurance covers them for both in-person and TMH practice. In addition, they may wish to consider policies on supervisor insurance coverage for e-supervision.

Handbooks. Standard 4.G specifies, "Programs provide a fieldwork handbook to all students and fieldwork site supervisors, for all program delivery types, detailing requirements, expectations, policies, and procedures." Counselor education program handbooks should include any policies on TMH or e-supervision and policies on data security of devices used for such services.

Supervisor qualifications. CACREP Standards 4.N through 4.P outline various requirements and qualifications for field placement supervisors and group/individual faculty supervisors. In this section, CACREP addresses TMH and e-supervision directly. Regarding individual or group supervision faculty, 4.N.2 requires they have "relevant training for in-person and/or distance counseling supervision," and 4.N.3 requires "relevant training in the technology utilized for supervision." Those same standards are required for site fieldwork supervisors in Standards 4.P.4 and 4.P.5. Thus, the counselor education program is responsible for ensuring that supervisors, including site and faculty supervisors who are offering TMH and e-supervision, have been trained in its use and appropriate technology. Finally, Standard 4.P.2 requires that fieldwork site supervisors have "active certifications and/or licenses in the geographic location where the student is placed." Counselor education programs must be designed with an awareness of TMH laws in their region to ensure that site supervisors supervising CITs in TMH are eligible to do so.

Fieldwork Seminar Instruction

Recordings. Standard 4.C requires that "supervision of practicum and internship students includes secure audio or video recordings and/or live supervision of students' interactions with clients that are in compliance with applicable institutional, state, federal, and international privacy requirements for all program delivery types." Counselor education programs must be aware of privacy and security issues impacting the recording, transmission, and storage of these sessions. Any risks need to be included in consent and release forms.

Counseling skills and activities. Standard 4.E states that students must engage in both group and individual counseling during either practicum or internship. CITs engaging in TMH group or individual counseling should have received training as addressed in Chapters 7 and 8. In addition, Standard 4.D specifies, "Students have the opportunity to become familiar with a variety of professional activities and resources, including technology, as part of their practicum and internship." Thus, CITs should be exposed to any relevant technology being used on-site.

Evaluations. In line with Standard 4.F, CITs should receive "formative and summative evaluations of the student's counseling performance and ability to integrate and apply knowledge are conducted as part of the student's practicum and internship." Counseling education programs may elect to adapt their formal evaluations to include an evaluation of TMH skills. In addition, students should have an opportunity to evaluate their site and supervisor (Standard 4.M), as well as their field placement process (Standard 4.L). These evaluations may also be adapted to include an evaluation of TMH training or TMH services provided by the site and supervisor or the information they were provided with during field placement on TMH options.

Communication With Supervisors

Successful fieldwork experiences include active dialogue between the counselor education program and the fieldwork site supervisor. University faculty communicate with fieldwork site supervisors in many ways, including before and during placement. CACREP specifies guidelines for this communication, which can also be adapted to include TMH practice and supervision.

Supervisor agreements and orientation. CACREP Standards 4.H.1–3 specify the content to be included in written supervision agreements, including the roles and responsibilities of the university supervisor and the field supervisor. If TMH or e-supervision is utilized at the site, these written agreements can be adapted to include specifications on TMH training and other policies. In addition, Standard 4.I specifies that "the counselor education program provides orientation to fieldwork site supervisors regarding program requirements and expectations." Like supervisor handbooks and agreements, the orientation should specify any standards or expectations regarding TMH and e-supervision.

Consultation and communication. Standard 4.G specifies that "the counselor education program engages in consultation with the fieldwork site supervisor to monitor student learning and performance in accordance with the supervision agreement." These communication and consultation sessions are often conducted via technology, including phone, email, or video, in addition to on-site visits. Counselor education programs need to consider how they document these communications and any specifications required to store and/or transmit virtual summaries of these consultation meetings.

Professional development training. Finally, Standard 4.K requires that "the counselor education program provides professional development opportunities to fieldwork site supervisors for all program delivery types." This standard provides an opportunity for counselor education programs to train supervisors should they lack TMH training or e-supervision training.

Other Considerations for Fieldwork Instruction

The CACREP standards support the inclusion of TMH into professional practice in ways beyond those outlined above. Specifically, CACREP ratios of 1:6 for doctoral student supervisors (Standard 4.Y) and 1:12 for counselor educator supervisors support using smaller ratios for e-supervision, as group supervision is ineffective with groups larger than 12 (4.BB). Similarly, CACREP requirements for both individual/triadic supervision (Standard 4.W) and group supervision (4.X) provide increased oversight for students in fieldwork. As TMH practice involves a variety of ethical practice concerns, students engaging in TMH during fieldwork will benefit from additional levels of supervision.

Fieldwork Techniques

I typically include teaching techniques at the end of each chapter, as well as suggested instructional strategies for integrating TMH into CIT coursework. Since fieldwork and professional practice involve the instruction of seminar courses, administration and planning, and communication with fieldwork site supervisors, I instead provide suggested counselor education program strategies on including TMH in these various programmatic elements.

1. *Student TMH Training.* Students who are expected to engage in TMH practice should have received training in TMH throughout their program or should receive TMH training from the fieldwork site. Sites engaging in TMH should train students in any software required to ethically and safely provide TMH services. Other training suggestions are included in Chapter 1, which can be recommended to supervisors. In addition, counselor education programs that systematically infuse TMH content throughout the generalized and specialized curricula will support CITs' success in using TMH with their clients and students.
2. *Supervisor Training.* Supervisors, whether site supervisors or faculty supervisors, need training in TMH (if CITs are engaging in TMH practice) and/or e-supervision if they are using distance supervision methods. The counselor education program can develop training programs focused on TMH or e-supervision.

Foundational TMH training resources are included in Chapter 1. E-supervision resources are available in Stretch et al. (2013) and Goss et al. (2016), specifically, "Part II, Use of Technology in Training and Supervision."

3. *Policies for TMH During Fieldwork.* Counselor education programs can develop policies regarding engaging in TMH during fieldwork. Such policies might include provisions on TMH access to the supervisor, TMH training, and not using personal devices for TMH practice. These policies should be outlined in both student and supervisor handbooks. Counselor education programs may wish to review other program handbooks for their policies on TMH and e-supervision.
4. *Recorded Counseling Sessions.* Fieldwork experience requires audio or video recordings of sessions or live supervision. For counselor education programs in which students record sessions, the program should create specific policies for the recording, storage, transmission, and disposal of any counseling videos, particularly for students engaging in TMH or supervisors utilizing e-supervision. Policies should consider data safety, security, encryption practices, and protocols should data be compromised.
5. *E-supervision.* Faculty supervisors with training in e-supervision can expose CITs to various models of e-supervision, including video and phone modalities, as well as text or chat, via individual/group/triadic formats. CITs can discuss the strengths and weaknesses of each model. Chapter 2 discusses the technological tools needed to conduct this practice.
6. *Video Reflection and Vlogging in Fieldwork.* Instructors can consider technological interventions to support fieldwork instruction and student reflection. Video journaling (Parikh et al., 2012) and vlogging (Brott & Willis, 2021) are two examples.
7. *Self-Assessment of TMH Skills.* CITs regularly self-assess their counseling skills during fieldwork experiences, utilizing tools such as the Counselor Activity Self Efficacy Scales (CASES; Lent et al., 2003) or the Counseling Self Estimate Inventory (COSE; Larson et al., 1992). For students engaging in TMH practice, instructors can adapt self-evaluation tools for CITs to assess their TMH skills compared to their in-person skills.
8. *TMH Emergency Procedures in Fieldwork.* A reality of counseling practice is the need to contact authorities in the event of emergencies, such as suicidal or homicidal intent, which can

be complicated by TMH delivery. Fieldwork instructors can specifically assign CITs to explore emergency procedures at their fieldwork site pertaining to emergency situations, such that they are aware of them before a situation arises (Robertson, 2013). This practice may reduce CITs' worry about these practices should they occur. CITs can report the policies in place to the class while maintaining the confidentiality of the site and/or clients/students.

9. *TMH Informed Consent.* CITs trained in TMH have been instructed that TMH informed consent documents include additional information beyond traditional informed consent documents. Instructors can advise CITs to examine the informed consent documents on their site and any references to TMH services. CITs can practice reviewing TMH informed consent with various clients, including adults, adolescents, and guardians, and explaining the essential elements of TMH counseling.
10. *Data Safety and Security.* CITs trained in TMH have been instructed that protocols and precautions must be maintained for data safety and security. CITs can inquire at their site about the data safety and security practices for TMH tools, such that they can explain these precautions to clients or guardians who inquire. CITs can report back to class the practices in place at their fieldwork site while maintaining the confidentiality of the site and/or clients/students.

19

Counselor Education and Supervision

Counselors-in-training (CITs) pursuing doctoral studies in counselor education and supervision (CES) often pursue post-graduation careers as university faculty in CES programs or as clinical supervisors. This book is written primarily for counselor educators and CES doctoral students who wish to infuse information on telemental health (TMH) counseling into their training of master's level counselors. Counselor Education and Supervision (CES) is included in Section 6 of the 2024 CACREP standards and includes information on the program, the doctoral curriculum, the doctoral internship, the doctoral counseling internship, and faculty course loads and ratios. Since this book focuses on the teaching of TMH, this chapter will focus on the doctoral curriculum and strategies for CES instructors to include TMH content in a doctoral curriculum.

CACREP Curriculum Standards

CACREP Standard 6 (Doctoral Standards for Counselor Education and Supervision) includes Section B (The Doctoral Curriculum), addressing educational standards in five areas: Counseling, Supervision, Teaching, Research/Scholarship, and Leadership/Advocacy. These five areas include nearly 60 educational standards pertaining to the doctoral curriculum. Some of these standards specifically address the use of technology in counseling practice. Tables 19.1 through 19.5 provide suggestions on how TMH content is connected to CACREP doctoral standards. If these concepts are unfamiliar, the instructor is reminded to explore the training and reading materials suggested in Chapter 1 and other chapters.

It should be noted that any of these topics could be addressed in a chapter or even an entire book instead of being reduced to a single table. Topics such as doctoral counseling, teaching, supervision, and research are often full-semester courses, if not multiple semesters. Thus, these tables provide a cursory view of the topic regarding including TMH content in doctoral instruction. It should also be noted that many of these topics could also serve as a focus of doctoral research aimed at the infusion of TMH into the doctoral curriculum, which will be addressed in the section Doctoral Research and Scholarship.

Doctoral Counseling

CACREP Standard 6.B.1 (Doctoral Counseling) identifies six curricular standards for doctoral CITs.

Table 19.1

CACREP Standard 6.B.1 (Doctoral Counseling) and Suggested TMH Content

CACREP Standards (2024)	Suggested TMH Content
6.B.1.a. Scholarly examination of the evidence base for counseling processes and theories.	Critical examination of the literature on TMH and its effectiveness with different populations and clinical issues spanning several decades to the present.
6.B.1.b. Integration of theories relevant to counseling.	Similar to 6.B.1.a, critical examination of the literature on theoretical approaches with evidence to support its use in TMH settings.
6.B.1.c. Conceptualization of clients from multiple theoretical perspectives.	Pros and cons of TMH for case conceptualization; similar to 6.B.1.b, crucial examining of literature on theoretical approaches and TMH use.

CACREP Standards (2024)	Suggested TMH Content
6.B.1.d. Scholarly examination of culturally sustaining counseling practice across multiple settings, contexts, and across service delivery modalities.	Expanding contexts from Chapter 4 and clinical chapters (Chapters 11, 13, & 14), examining TMH with different cultural communities, treatment settings, and contexts. "Across service delivery modalities" implies TMH via multiple modalities (e.g., phone, video) and in-person counseling
6.B.1.e. Methods for evaluating counseling effectiveness.	Expanding on program evaluation content from Chapter 10, evaluating TMH services and examining research based on TMH effectiveness.
6.B.1.f. Legal and ethical issues and responsibilities in counseling across multiple settings and across service delivery modalities	Tools to remain current on legal and ethical issues pertaining to TMH; ability to train master's students on accessing timely information on TMH laws and ethics.

Doctoral Supervision

Doctoral studies involve training in supervision. Online supervision, or e-supervision, has been addressed in professional literature. Several metanalyses have examined research related to online supervision and identified common factors that both support and hinder effective supervision (Inman et al., 2019; Martin et al., 2018; Phillips et al., 2021). Sheperis and Sadeh-Sharvit (2023) argue that artificial intelligence (AI) can substantially benefit the supervision experience and advocate for AI simulation-based training clinics and voice–tone recognition software to identify CITs' emotions during recorded sessions. In one study, supervisors had a positive attitude about AI's potential for professional growth yet questioned its ability to evaluate issues such as rapport, culture, and nonverbal communication. Simultaneously, clinicians expressed concerns about their confidentiality should they receive low supervision ratings (Creed et al., 2022). Instructors training CES CITs in supervision will need to include content on e-supervision as the practice continues to grow. CACREP Standard 6.B.2 (Doctoral Supervision) identifies twelve curricular standards for doctoral CITs.

Table 19.2

CACREP Standard 6.B.2 (Doctoral Supervision) and Suggested TMH Content

CACREP Standards (2024)	Suggested TMH Content
6.B.2.a. Purposes of counseling supervision.	Purposes of e-supervision; urgency and need for e-supervision with the increase in TMH provision.
6.B.2.b. Theoretical frameworks and models of counseling supervision.	Applying supervision models and frameworks to TMH/e-supervision practices.
6.B.2.c. Roles and relationships related to counseling supervision.	Examining the supervisor/supervisee relationship between e-supervision and in-person supervision; examining the supervisee/supervisor relationship for AI supervision; technology power and privilege in supervision (Singh et al., 2020).
6.B.2.d. Skills of counseling supervision across multiple settings and across service delivery modalities.	Like TMH, translating supervisory skills and techniques to e-supervision settings (e.g., school, addictions) and modalities (e.g., phone, video).
6.B.2.e. Opportunities for developing a personal style of counseling supervision grounded in theory and research.	Adaptations to personal supervision style for e-supervision.
6.B.2.f. Assessment of supervisees' developmental level and other relevant characteristics.	Assessing supervisees from a distance; Digital observation; safety of data storage and transmission of supervisee tapes or transcripts; pros and cons of using AI to support supervisee assessment.
6.B.2.g. Modalities of counseling supervision, including individual, triadic, and group supervision.	Similar to 6.B.2.b, applying supervision modalities to TMH/e-supervision practices.
6.B.2.h The use of technology in counseling supervision.	Practice of e-supervision; emergency e-supervision; technology utilized to support supervision, e.g., documentation, email.

CACREP Standards (2024)	Suggested TMH Content
6.B.2.i. Administrative procedures and responsibilities related to counseling supervision.	Adapting administrative procedures to digital forums, e.g., documentation, recordings, notes, transmission of data; importance of data security for e-supervision practice.
6.B.2.j. Evaluation, remediation, and gatekeeping in counseling supervision.	Capacity for e-supervision to support remediation practices, including observation and access to supervisees' sessions.
6.B.2.k. Legal and ethical issues and responsibilities in counseling supervision.	Ethical framework for using technology in supervision (Stretch et al., 2013).
6.B.2.l. Culturally sustaining strategies for conducting counseling supervision	The benefits/risks of e-supervision mirror those of TMH, including access to diverse supervisors with varying clinical expertise while also creating potential obstacles due to the digital divide.

Doctoral Teaching

I have shared how this book is written primarily for counselor educators and CES doctoral students to infuse information on telemental health (TMH) counseling into master's level training. CES programs and faculty are also charged with providing doctoral CITs information on the teaching and training of master's students. Much of this book aims to support master's level faculty in their TMH teaching techniques. In Chapter 2, I discuss the various teaching modalities (e.g., online, on campus) where TMH training may occur. Due to this earlier foundation, in this chapter, I'll briefly reinforce how concepts of TMH can be integrated into doctoral coursework and how TMH can be infused into various teaching modalities. CACREP Standard 6.B.3 (Doctoral Teaching) identifies thirteen curricular standards for doctoral CIT.

Table 19.3

CACREP Standard 6.B.3 (Doctoral Teaching) and Suggested TMH Content

CACREP Standards (2024)	Suggested TMH Content
6.B.3.a. Roles and responsibilities related to educating counselors.	The responsibility of counselor educators to train CIT in TMH as practice expands.
6.B.3.b. Andragogy and adult learning theories.	Concepts of adult learning as they pertain to TMH instruction, including self-motivated learning, using prior experiences, recognizing a need for information, and immediately applying learning in real world context (Knowles, 1975). See "Teaching Techniques" in each chapter.
6.B.3.c. Teaching methods relevant to counselor education.	Like TMH, various CES instructional methods meet the needs of students, whether in person or online.
6.B.3.d. Curriculum design and instructional delivery.	Integrating TMH into counseling curricula (see Sections 2 and 3 of this book); wide variety of online teaching tools (e.g., learning management systems (LMS), survey tools) to support both online and face-to-face (F2F) instruction.
6.B.3.e. The use of technology in instructional design and program delivery types.	Like 6.B.3.d, integrating TMH into curriculum; using technology appropriately and effectively within CIT training; awareness of federal standards surrounding third-party platforms in higher education (U.S. Department of Education, 2023).
6.B.3.f. Integration of diversity, equity, inclusion, and social justice principles and practices in the counselor education curriculum.	Reinforcing capacity for TMH to support access and equity issues only if technology is accessible to client and student populations (see Chapters 4, 14, and 15).

CACREP Standards (2024)	Suggested TMH Content
6.B.3.g. Universal design to meet the needs of all students with respect for individual differences in learning.	Like TMH, the capacity for technology to support universal design for CITs if accessible and compliant with the Americans with Disabilities Act (ADA) (see Chapter 14).
6.B.3.h. Instructional and curricular evaluation methods.	Adapting instruction and curriculum to include didactic and experiential TMH learning.
6.B.3.i. Screening, remediation, and gatekeeping functions relevant to teaching.	Challenges in screening distance students; capacity for e-supervision to support remediation practices, including observation and access to supervisee sessions; risks of engaging in TMH for CITs with remote clients and supervisors.
6.B.3.j. Assessment of student learning and professional dispositions.	Challenges in screening distance students; TMH practice to reinforce content from Chapter 9 for challenges in online assessment.
6.B.3.k. Legal and ethical issues and responsibilities in counselor education for all program delivery types.	Legal and ethical issues, as well as institutional policies, in TMH and distance teaching; reinforcing content from Chapter 3 for ethical/legal issues in TMH, and ethical issues in e-supervision (Stretch et al., 2013).
6.B.3.l. Culturally sustaining strategies for counselor education	Reinforcing capacity for TMH to support access and equity issues, if accessible to client and student population (see Chapter 4).
6.B.3.m. The role of mentoring in counselor education.	Importance of modeling, supervision, and mentorship in both teaching and counseling practice; including modeling of TMH, e-supervision, and online instruction.

Doctoral Research and Scholarship

Master's level counselors receive instruction in research and program evaluation as outlined in Chapter 10. While some master's programs may utilize a thesis model, most master's programs are not preparing

CITs to be researchers but to be professional counselors. At the doctoral level, however, CITs are expected to engage in original research as a component of their doctoral dissertation. Thus, doctoral CITs are trained in more advanced and varied research approaches than during their master's studies. Integrating TMH into doctoral research instruction can take many forms, including examining the literature for trends in TMH concepts or conducting one's own research on TMH. In Chapter 10, I discuss conducting research online, whereas, in this chapter, I'll suggest some of those concepts but also introduce the prospect of examining TMH as a focus of one's research agenda. CACREP Standard 6.B.4 (Doctoral Research and Scholarship) identifies thirteen curricular standards for doctoral CITs.

Table 19.4

CACREP Standard 6.B.4 (Doctoral Research and Scholarship) and Suggested TMH Content

CACREP Standards (2024)	Suggested TMH Content
6.B.4.a Research designs appropriate to quantitative, qualitative, mixed methods, and action research questions or hypotheses.	Considering varied research designs, questions, and hypotheses that will expand the research base and knowledge regarding the efficacy of TMH.
6.B.4.b. Quantitative data analysis methods.	Capacity for online statistical software to support data analysis for both online and in-person research.
6.B.4.c. Qualitative approaches to data analysis.	Capacity for video/phone recording platforms to support online interviews and observations as needed for qualitative methods; additional software tools available to support qualitative data analysis (e.g., transcript evaluations).
6.B.4.d. Models and methods of sampling relevant to research design.	Capacity for online research to expand access to respondents; limitations of online research pertaining to digital access of potential respondents.

CACREP Standards (2024)	Suggested TMH Content
6.B.4.e. Models and methods of instrument design.	The need to validate assessment instruments for online administration as a component of instrument design or to develop a literature base on the online administration of assessment instruments (see Chapter 9).
6.B.4.f. Models and methods of program evaluation.	Adapting program evaluation models for TMH delivery; importance of evaluating online TMH services.
6.B.4.g. Research questions or hypotheses appropriate for professional research and publication.	Examining the TMH literature for gaps and identifying research questions or studies to fill TMH gaps in the literature.
6.B.4.h. Professional writing for peer-reviewed journal publication.	Seeking professional journals focusing on research highlighting technology in counselor education, e.g., the *Journal of Technology in Counselor Education and Supervision* (JTCES).
6.B.4.i. Professional conference proposal preparation.	Identifying professional conferences that highlight the use of technology and distance practices, e.g., Counselor Education Distance Learning conference at Palo Alto University.
6.B.4.j. Development of research proposals for a human subjects/institutional review board review.	Emphasis on research data security and data storage for online research or research focused on TMH, as required by institutional review boards (IRB). Practice outlining data security procedures for IRB proposals.
6.B.4.k. Grant proposals and other sources of funding.	Identifying how TMH can fill service gaps for needed communities and seeking grant opportunities supporting research with TMH approaches.
6.B.4.l. Strategies for conducting culturally relevant and culturally competent research.	Capacity for online research to expand the pool of respondents; limitations of online research pertaining to digital access of potential respondents.

CACREP Standards (2024)	Suggested TMH Content
6.B.4.m. Ethical considerations and strategies for conducting research.	ACA Code of Ethics (2014) Sections G (Research and Publication) and H (Distance Counseling), as well as specialization codes, such as those of ASCA, AMHCA, NCDA, and NAADAC.

Doctoral Leadership and Advocacy

Doctoral-level CITs often assume leadership positions within the counseling profession. Like all professional counselors, counselor educators, supervisors, and doctoral students are expected to advocate for the counseling profession and the clients and students they serve. While counselor educators, supervisors, and doctoral CITs may advocate for various professional or clinical issues, they may also advocate for the ethical and effective use of TMH within the profession. CACREP Standard 6.B.5 (Doctoral Leadership and Advocacy) identify fourteen curricular standards for doctoral CITs.

Table 19.5

CACREP Standard 6.B.5 (Doctoral Leadership and Advocacy) and Suggested TMH Content

CACREP Standards (2024)	Suggested TMH Related Concepts
CACREP Standards (2024)	Suggested TMH Related Concepts
6.B.5.a. Theories, models, and skills of leadership.	Variations in leadership theories, models, and skills when serving as an online leader.
6.B.5.b. Leadership and leadership development in professional organizations.	Professional organization interest groups focused on technology or TMH, e.g., ACA Member Interest Communities: Counseling and Technology Interest Network, Artificial Intelligence Interest Network, Distance Learning in Counselor Education.

CACREP Standards (2024)	Suggested TMH Related Concepts
6.B.5.c. Leadership in counselor education programs.	Role of department leaders to bring emerging trends to programs to remain current, such as TMH, AI, and other advances in technology.
6.B.5.d. Accreditation standards and program accreditation processes, including self-studies and program reports.	Infusing TMH into CACREP accreditation general curriculum and specialization standards (see Sections 2 and 3 of this book).
6.B.5.e. Management and administration in agencies, organizations, and other institutions.	Models of administration for online, in-person, and hybrid organizations, institutions, or agencies. Modeling effective TMH practice and supervision within organizations and agencies.
6.B.5.f. Leadership roles and strategies for responding to crises and disasters.	Value of on-ground leadership/strategies versus online leadership/strategies during crises and disasters.
6.B.5.g. Strategies of leadership in consultation.	Distance consultation strategies.
6.B.5.h. Current sociopolitical and social justice issues and how those issues affect the counseling profession.	Capacity for TMH to serve marginalized and targeted groups impacted by sociopolitical and social justice issues, coupled with the reality of digital inequities and infrastructure limitations.
6.B.5.i. Models and competencies for counselors and counselor educators advocating on behalf of the profession and professional counselor identity.	Variations in advocacy models and competencies when serving as an online advocate.
6.B.5.j. Models and competencies for advocating for clients at the individual, system, and policy levels.	Advocacy for access to technology and reducing the digital divide; advocacy for infrastructure improvements, technology training, insurance coverage for TMH, etc.

CACREP Standards (2024)	Suggested TMH Related Concepts
6.B.5.k. Strategies of leadership in relation to diversity, equity, inclusion, and social justice issues.	Capacity for leaders to recognize inequities in accessing counseling services, which may include TMH services, and taking action to address issues of equity, inclusion, and social justice.
6.B.5.l. Culturally sustaining leadership and advocacy practices.	Importance of leading and advocating within cultural communities versus on behalf of them. The risks of TMH and online leadership/advocacy to remove the in-person access and live observation of various cultural communities.
6.B.5.n. Role of self-care in advocacy and leadership.	Capacity for online roles (e.g., leadership, advocacy, counseling, teaching) to blur lines of professional and personal boundaries—increasing capacity for burnout. Importance of maintaining self-care when engaging in TMH and online practices.

Teaching Techniques

Sample teaching techniques are included below since this chapter has not included doctoral lessons. The strategies below support the instruction of TMH within the doctoral curricula, using andragogical principles, including self-motivated learning, using prior experiences, recognizing a need for information, and immediately applying learning in a real-world context (Knowles, 1975).

1. *Counseling: TMH Efficacy.* Doctoral CITs are encouraged to examine TMH literature for efficacy studies in clinical practice. CITs are encouraged to seek out efficacy studies on various clinical foci, clients/student populations, and issues. CITs can compare and contrast earlier literature findings on TMH with more recent studies, including carefully examining pre- and post-COVID-19 research.
2. *Counseling: Evaluating TMH Counseling Effectiveness.* Instructors and doctoral CITs can explore various methods of evaluating

TMH counseling effectiveness, including achievement of client/student goals, client/student surveys, and other strategies. CITs and instructors can discuss how TMH practice may impact counseling effectiveness.

3. *Supervision: Supervisory relationships.* Doctoral CITs can explore the e-supervision supervisee-supervisor relationship. CITs and instructors can discuss supervisor characteristics needed in e-supervision to support and sustain the virtual relationship and how these characteristics may vary from in-person supervision, if at all.
4. *Supervision: E-supervision and remediation.* Doctoral students can discuss and debate the pros and cons of e-supervision in counselor coaching and remediation. What elements of e-supervision are supported by virtual relationships, and which are at risk?
5. *Teaching Internship:* Many doctoral CITs complete a teaching internship within their program or teach lessons in master's courses as a component of their training. CITs can be instructed to adapt one of the lessons used in their doctoral teaching internship to include content on TMH. Using the strategies discussed in Chapter 2, doctoral CITs can create opportunities for master's students to practice TMH and apply their learning to mock sessions. Instructors provide feedback on the adaptation of the lesson and the impact on students.
6. *Teaching:* Doctoral CITs can be instructed to select one of the sample lessons in Sections 2 and 3 of this book focused on integrating TMH content into a curricular area. Doctoral CITs can practice delivering the lesson on TMH in multiple classroom formats, including on-campus, online synchronous, and online synchronous to various audiences. The instructor and/or doctoral peers can provide feedback on CIT teaching style and student impact.
7. *Research: Identifying TMH Research Gaps.* Doctoral CITs can comprehensively review TMH literature pertaining to a particular TMH construct (e.g., access, effectiveness, client satisfaction). CITs should identify gaps in the literature that have not been adequately addressed in the literature.
8. *Research: Developing TMH Research Questions.* Expanding on the literature search conducted in item 7, CITs can develop research questions and/or hypotheses that address aspects of TMH literature that are scarce.

9. *Advocacy: Considering the Counseling Compact.* Many states are advocating for the Counseling Compact to expand access to counseling services for clients and counselors alike. Yet, some states are concerned that reimbursement rates in different states will negatively impact counselor income and/or competition. CITs and instructors can discuss and debate the Counseling Compact as an equity access tool, including both counselor and client advocacy.
10. *Leadership: Online Leadership.* Doctoral CITs can research one leadership role in the counseling profession and explore both the online and in-person commitment of the position. Doctoral CITs can share their findings in class, discussing the benefits and challenges of these leadership positions as well as incorporating their own wellness and self-care as they consider various leadership roles. Doctoral CITs can develop wellness plans to minimize blurring the boundaries between online work and their personal lives.

20

The Future of Telemental Health Counseling and Training

We have all heard the phrase, "The future is now." The origins of that phrase have been credited to all manner of sources, including novelists, documentaries, and football coaches. Yet, regarding telemental health (TMH) counseling, the phrase's origin is less important than its context. The context is that many of the concepts discussed in this chapter are happening right now instead of in the future. This chapter describes emerging trends in TMH counseling and training. Some topics were mentioned in other chapters of the book, yet not extensively, because of the relative novelty of the practice, its limited present use, or lack of research on TMH as it relates to the counseling profession. Nothing in this chapter will be new or unknown to most readers. Some readers may adapt these concepts into their practice, while others are less familiar or comfortable with the trends. It is expected, however, that their use will expand in the future.

I concede that the future includes systems and strategies as yet unknown. It is unlikely that any of us would have predicted the widespread use of TMH without the COVID-19 pandemic propelling us fully into TMH practice. Many counselor educators met with student opposition to TMH practice during the COVID-19 pandemic. I remember one student pleading to me, "This is not what I wanted to do, Dr. Robertson.

This is not why I wanted to become a counselor," when she learned she would be expected to practice via TMH. Even those of us who studied and researched TMH before the pandemic were met with resistance. In another instance, following a TMH grant I received in 2016, a senior colleague and supervisor told me, "I don't like it, and I don't think we should do it," regarding my research on TMH training and practice. These statements echoed earlier opposition to distance education and those who opposed training counselors via distance technology. Yet colleagues have changed their minds. I cannot predict the future with any certainty for TMH, but the future is now. And the only sure thing is change.

TMH Counseling

Virtual Reality (VR)

I begin with virtual reality (VR), the oldest "emerging" technology in TMH. Often used as a type of exposure therapy, wide-use empirical research on VR is limited, although small-scale and single-subject research exists. There is a rich history of VR and its infusion into multiple industries, including education and counseling. Raja and Lakshmi Priya (2021) present a historical timeline of VR, dating back to 1838 as a conceptual model and citing a 1929 flight simulator as one of its first practices. Citing Sherman and Craig (2018), Raja and Lakshmi Priya present the key elements of virtual reality, including a virtual world, immersion, sensory feedback, and interactivity (p. 118).

VR involves sight, sound, and sometimes tactile, physical, and olfactory immersion experiences. These simulations mimic stress-inducing or calm-inducing scenarios. Users are often coached/trained by counselors to practice skills learned in either TMH or in-person sessions during these VR simulations. The benefit of VR simulation in counseling is that it recreates situations in a safe and supportive setting and allows the client to practice skills learned in therapy before encountering those situations in the real world. Some examples of VR involve simulations for phobias, trauma, and posttraumatic stress disorder (PTSD; Hofstra University, n.d.), contamination-related obsessive-compulsive disorders (OCD; Miegel et al., 2022), and cravings for persons with alcohol use disorder (AUD; Lütt et al., 2023).

Several clinics and counseling settings use VR; however, the cost of such technologies and the training of clinicians limit its use. As these technologies become more user-friendly and affordable, we can expect to see an increase in training and use of VR in counseling, including

TMH counseling. One challenge of using VR in TMH settings relates to the clinician's limited control over the client's setting, which may need to be controlled for effective treatment. While the clinician can set expectations, using VR simulations can be risky when a client is not physically located in the same space as the counselor, particularly for simulations invoking trauma or phobia responses. Should a VR simulation session trigger harmful or dangerous behavior in the client, the counselor must ensure client safety. Another challenge is ensuring that the client can access the technology for VR experiences in a remote setting. As with TMH, these tools may become more affordable as technology advances.

Artificial Intelligence (AI)

Artificial intelligence (AI) gained wide attention in 2022 and 2023, with increased focus on the use of ChatGPT and OpenAI. The chatbot technology utilized in ChatGPT was not new. "Virtual assistants" have been present on many online platforms, from online retail sites to university websites. A historical view of GPT (generative pretrained transformer) described GPT-1 being introduced in 2018, followed by GPT-2 in 2019, and GPT-3 in 2020. Yet the improvements to GPT-4 and the use of ChatGPT displayed more humanistic-type traits, including its ability to "follow the user's intention," "lower likelihood of dangerous or offensive output," increased accuracy, and more "steerability," meaning its ability to adapt based on the user's request (Marr, 2023, para. 13).

The use of AI in counseling and mental health treatment is also not new. AI has been used in diagnosing mental health conditions and developing treatment plans. Electronic medical record (EMR) systems have long been able to summarize information entered by a clinician into a client's record, produce a recommended clinical diagnosis, and write a clinical summary of the intake. These EMR programs can utilize intake and clinical diagnosis data to recommend treatment plan goals and objectives. These tools are not meant to replace clinicians; on the contrary, several have built-in safeguards to ensure that the clinician reviews and edits the suggested outcomes. However, they are designed to reduce the workload of clinicians and minimize human error, such as ensuring that essential information is included. These tools require a human element to enter data into the system and generate the report.

Newer tools, such as Freed.AI, offer services in recording client/patient sessions and then generating SOAP (subjective, objective, assessment, and plan; Cameron & Turtle-Song, 2002) notes on behalf of the clinician (Freed, 2023a). There is a concern that a clinician may be sacrificing the confidentiality of client sessions by allowing recording, storage, and analysis of client sessions in a third-party platform. While the platform posts a public privacy and security statement (Freed, 2023b), questions arise regarding who owns the data entered into the system. More than a transcription service, these technologies review and analyze the content of these sessions, including confidential information, to create notes. Similar platforms are likely to emerge or already exist.

AI has advanced beyond generating language to generating images and media. These developments have triggered discussions about the ability of AI to replace humans in several work settings. The newest AI versions simulate human expression and perceive human intent, causing people to question if AI will replace human service workers and medical professionals. The amount of mental health and medical information from reputable online sources has already reduced reliance on such professionals. AI has eliminated pretreatment interventions through screening tools (Kister et al., 2023) and EMRs discussed above. But not without risks.

National Public Radio (NPR) highlighted a story in which the National Eating Disorders Association (NEDA) implemented a chatbot hotline in response to the large volume of calls that the human-staffed hotline experienced during and post-COVID-19 (Wells, 2023). The system eventually began providing weight loss information in response to texts from callers—dangerous advice for eating disorder callers. While the AI hotline was taken down when the problem was identified, NEDA had unfortunately disbanded its human-staffed hotline with the inception of the chatline. It's important to note that the chatline was initially created by eating disorders specialists with limited data responses. However, in one of its updates, the company that operates the chatline "added generative artificial intelligence, meaning it gave [the chatline] the ability to learn from new data and generate new responses" (Wells, 2023, para. 17). The NEDA example is one in which even the best-planned intentions (e.g., eating disorder specialists creating a chatbot with limited response to minimize risks created) can go awry.

Other examples beyond chatbots and report generation include using **avatars** to provide virtual counseling using AI responses. Much like digisexualities (McArthur & Twist, 2017), these digital personas may be comforting and less threatening than interacting with human clinicians for some people. How counselors utilize AI in their TMH practice has yet to be seen. Using digital avatars lends itself to TMH practice, where digital communication is already being used. However, counselors must balance the risk of such technologies with their primary ethical responsibility to protect client welfare.

Mobile Apps

Mobile applications, more commonly known as "apps," typically refer to programs downloadable to mobile devices such as smartphones or tablets. **Mobile apps**, like VR and AI, have been in place since the invention of the mobile phone. Some mobile apps are a compliment to an online website. Still, other sites are only accessible via the mobile app. Mobile apps have been used to reduce waiting time to access counseling treatment (Epstein & Bequette, 2013; Haeger et al., 2022). Mobile apps may complement counseling treatment (either TMH or in-person counseling) or be used as a stand-alone tool, sometimes at a counselor's or counseling website's recommendation. They may be used in TMH or face-to-face (F2F) counseling equally, although TMH settings may implicitly promote the use of technology in treatment.

Apps used to track and monitor mental health systems are introduced daily. Mental health mobile app developers are encouraged to create positive ratings for their products, like any other business or product. It is the monetization of mental health treatment as a business or product that raises concerns about promoting mental health apps in counseling. Mental and medical healthcare is certainly a business—no one will deny that (at least not in the United States)—but it is balancing the business need with the ethical need to protect the client that garners concern. Data collection, storage, and usage are primary concerns when utilizing mobile apps.

Wearable technology, such as smartwatches, wrist/ankle bands, and heart monitors, capture health information like sleep patterns, breathing patterns, heart rate, substance use, and speech patterns. Ingestible digital tablets can monitor and transmit medical information to mobile phones used to administer medication (Trafton, 2018) or monitor medication compliance. This data may be confidential medical information protected under the Health Insurance Portability and Accountability Act (HIPAA). As a counselor, having real-time information/data on a client's symptomology could be more beneficial than relying on client self-report. However, reliance on self-report data allows the counselor to meet the client where they are based on the client's comfort. Once again, when using or recommending mobile apps, counselors must conduct a thorough risk analysis of the technology, using the APA App Evaluation Model (2024) and other tools to maximize client safety over clinical convenience.

Data Mining

Data mining is a topic well beyond the scope of this text but bears mentioning in a discussion of TMH. TMH counseling platforms include videoconferencing systems, telephone systems, email and chat systems, computer software, mobile apps, data storage, and EMR systems. These technologies, as well as cloud storage, create an opportunity for the data to be collected, breached, used, or sold by someone beyond the counselor or the client. The analysis and use of any large data set is a common and growing practice. Data mining and analysis are regularly utilized to examine the data from text-based crisis hotlines and occasionally to evaluate word utterances using AI in hotline phone calls (Medina Greenspan et al., 2023). The primary goal of these analyses is to improve services. Within our digital society, it is largely expected that any time we utilize a third-party system or software (e.g., social media sites) or download a mobile app, the creator of that system or application has access to our information. There are certainly settings where users control access to their data and what information is accessed, as well as lengthy term agreements concerning these platforms. However, the most secure method is simply not using the system, which is difficult in our technological era.

How data mining practices will shape the counseling profession and TMH has yet to be seen. Future clients may become so comfortable with these data mining activities that the warnings become innocuous. Conversely, as identity theft and data breaches grow and negatively affect the public, clients may become less eager to utilize these systems. Just as people learned of the risks of tobacco or fad-diet products and discontinued their use, so might this be the case with data mining. People will stop using tools that eventually cause them harm. Still, another outcome could be the development of improved technology that minimizes risk while maximizing security and convenience. Until that day, CITs learning to use these platforms will need to understand, accept, and explain to their clients that data mining is part of the package.

TMH Training

Training in Technological Tools and Interventions

Most doctoral programs in Counselor Education require applicants to have some counseling experience or certification/licensure in counseling gained through counseling experience. Since many counselor education programs train individuals who will become faculty in the field, it is logical that they seek candidates who have experience in counseling to train the next generation of counselors. Much like you would want a flight instructor to have flown a plane before teaching a pilot to fly one, we want counselor educators and instructors to have practice, if not expertise, in counseling before they train others. As VR, AI, mobile apps, and data mining practices become more common in TMH, those training the next generation of counselors will need to be well-versed in these technologies and their application to counseling. While not all instructors can maintain a counseling practice, engaging in TMH counseling is an excellent strategy for remaining current in the field and knowledgeable of best practices.

The concept of lifelong learning applies to instructors as well. As AI, VR, and other technologies grow in practice, instructors will need to expand their knowledge and skills in these areas. Some areas, like VR exposure therapy, may develop as a clinical specialization and be used only by skilled and trained clinicians with access to specific technology (e.g., biofeedback). Still others, such as mobile apps, AI, and data mining, will likely find their way into everyday use. Our responsibility to CITs is to share current, relevant, evidence-based counseling interventions as these practices solidify their place in the profession. This may require instructors to gain future training in using these tools. It may also require counselor educators to engage in research that broadens our evidence base for using these tools for ethical and effective practice.

Using AI to Train Counselors

Earlier in the chapter, I discussed the concerns about AI replacing counselors and other human services professionals, but these concerns also extend to instructors who train CITs. There are 132 fully online Counselor Education CACREP accredited programs as of December of 2023, including doctoral and master's programs in all CACREP specializations (e.g., school, mental health, addictions, rehabilitation, marriage/couples/family, student affairs, and career counseling). Thus, many instructors already use technology with CITs by providing instruction via synchronous and asynchronous learning. However, the extent to which AI is being used to train future counselors is not yet known.

Counselor educators may balk at AI, avatars, or nonhuman interactions being used to train counseling, which is, at its core, a human exchange. Yet most of us have engaged in simulated training environments for other topics. Those of us who work in university settings may have participated in active shooter or sexual harassment training that requires us to interact with an avatar and select a response based on what we have witnessed during the training. Even within the counseling profession, software products have emerged that allow CITs to view counseling scenarios and then record or select the best response based on the skills being used.

Some organizations are effectively utilizing AI in their counselor training. The Trevor Project, whose mission is to end suicide among lesbian, gay, bisexual, transgender, questioning, and queer young people, uses a Crisis Contact Simulator as part of its training for crisis hotline workers. Workers engage with digital personas who portray issues presented by various callers. Trevor Project's Head of AI and Engineering states:

> [The] simulator can engage in a prolonged back-and-forth dialogue with trainees. It can use language in the same way people do, including language LGBTQ youth often use to describe their experiences and emotions. The simulator maintains a consistent emotional and experiential narrative in talking about real-life feelings and situations. (Sparks, 2021, para. 3)

Using AI technology, simulators like the one described by the Trevor Project can reduce training time and costs. These simulators may be more effective than watching recordings of counseling sessions and more cost-effective than paying for live simulations (e.g., actors or student actors) to engage students in practice. As professional organizations use AI as part of their training programs, it stands to reason that educational organizations, such as universities, will follow suit. The Trevor Project states that many crisis counselors work evenings and weekends, creating a demand for training outside business hours. The simulation tool helps to meet that demand (Sparks, 2021). In text-based crisis settings, crisis workers may be working with up to nine callers/texters at one time, including people expressing thoughts of suicide (Medina Greenspan et al., 2023), emphasizing the importance of practicing their clinical skills in a safe setting, using AI-generated personas. Many educational institutions are experiencing increased preference for online and on-demand training, which can be met by infusing AI into instructional strategies.

Conclusion

The future of TMH counseling and training is here, and it will continue to expand. The practice and teaching of TMH utilize tools such as VR, AI, apps, and data mining to achieve its goal. As instructors, we need to stay current with these technologies to train future counselors in effective TMH practice. Yet, we can also explore how we can utilize these technologies to expand our own teaching and training programs. It is unlikely that any of these practices will dissolve completely. They will likely grow and evolve, perhaps including increased security measures. The technology we use to provide TMH may change, as may the technology we use to train future TMH counselors. Regardless of these changes, our commitment to ethical, evidence-based, and safe practices for our clients and students must remain.

Appendix A

ACA & NBCC Codes of Ethics on Telemental Health

American Counseling Association (ACA) Code of Ethics (2014)

Section H: Distance Counseling, Technology, and Social Media

Introduction

Counselors understand that the profession of counseling may no longer be limited to in-person, face-to-face interactions. Counselors actively attempt to understand the evolving nature of the profession with regard to distance counseling, technology, and social media and how such resources may be used to better serve their clients. Counselors strive to become knowledgeable about these resources. Counselors understand the additional concerns related to the use of distance counseling, technology, and social media and make every attempt to protect confidentiality and meet any legal and ethical requirements for the use of such resources.

H.1. Knowledge and Legal Considerations

H.1.a. Knowledge and Competency

Counselors who engage in the use of distance counseling, technology, and/or social media develop knowledge and skills regarding related technical, ethical, and legal considerations (e.g., special certifications, additional course work).

H.1.b. Laws and Statutes

Counselors who engage in the use of distance counseling, technology, and social media within their counseling practice understand that they may be subject to laws and regulations of both the counselor's practicing location and the client's place of residence. Counselors ensure that their clients are aware of pertinent legal rights and limitations governing the practice of counseling across state lines or international boundaries.

H.2. Informed Consent and Security

H.2.a. Informed Consent and Disclosure

Clients have the freedom to choose whether to use distance counseling, social media, and/or technology within the counseling process. In addition to the usual and customary protocol of informed consent between counselor and client for face-to-face counseling, the following issues, unique to the use of distance counseling, technology, and/ or social media, are addressed in the informed consent process:

- distance counseling credentials, physical location of practice, and contact information;
- risks and benefits of engaging in the use of distance counseling, technology, and/or social media;
- possibility of technology failure and alternate methods of service delivery;
- anticipated response time;
- emergency procedures to follow when the counselor is not available;
- time zone differences;
- cultural and/or language differences that may affect delivery of services;
- possible denial of insurance benefits; and
- social media policy.

H.2.b. Confidentiality Maintained by the Counselor

Counselors acknowledge the limitations of maintaining the confidentiality of electronic records and transmissions. They inform clients that individuals might have authorized or unauthorized access to such records or transmissions (e.g., colleagues, supervisors, employees, information technologists).

H.2.c. Acknowledgment of Limitations

Counselors inform clients about the inherent limits of confidentiality when using technology. Counselors urge clients to be aware of authorized and/or unauthorized access to information disclosed using this medium in the counseling process.

H.2.d. Security

Counselors use current encryption standards within their websites and/or technology-based communications that meet applicable legal requirements. Counselors take reasonable precautions to ensure the confidentiality of information transmitted through any electronic means.

H.3. Client Verification

Counselors who engage in the use of distance counseling, technology, and/or social media to interact with clients take steps to verify the client's identity at the beginning and throughout the therapeutic process. Verification can include, but is not limited to, using code words, numbers, graphics, or other nondescript identifiers.

H.4. Distance Counseling Relationship

H.4.a. Benefits and Limitations

Counselors inform clients of the benefits and limitations of using technology applications in the provision of counseling services. Such technologies include, but are not limited to, computer hardware and/or software, telephones and applications, social media and Internet-based applications and other audio and/or video communication, or data storage devices or media.

H.4.b. Professional Boundaries in Distance Counseling

Counselors understand the necessity of maintaining a professional relationship with their clients. Counselors discuss and establish professional boundaries with clients regarding the appropriate use and/or application of technology and the limitations of its use within the counseling relationship (e.g., lack of confidentiality, times when not appropriate to use).

H.4.c. Technology-Assisted Services

When providing technology-assisted services, counselors make reasonable efforts to determine that clients are intellectually, emotionally, physically, linguistically, and functionally capable of using the application and that the application is appropriate for the needs of the client. Counselors verify that clients understand the purpose and operation of technology applications and follow up with clients to correct possible misconceptions, discover appropriate use, and assess subsequent steps.

H.4.d. Effectiveness of Services

When distance counseling services are deemed ineffective by the counselor or client, counselors consider delivering services face-to-face. If the counselor is not able to provide face-to-face services (e.g., lives in another state), the counselor assists the client in identifying appropriate services.

H.4.e. Access

Counselors provide information to clients regarding reasonable access to pertinent applications when providing technology-assisted services

H.4.f. Communication Differences in Electronic Media

Counselors consider the differences between face-to-face and electronic communication (nonverbal and verbal cues) and how these may affect the counseling process. Counselors educate clients on how to prevent and address potential misunderstandings arising from the lack of visual cues and voice intonations when communicating electronically.

H.5. Records and Web Maintenance

H.5.a. Records

Counselors maintain electronic records in accordance with relevant laws and statutes. Counselors inform clients on how records are maintained electronically. This includes, but is not limited to, the type of encryption and security assigned to the records, and if/for how long archival storage of transaction records is maintained.

H.5.b. Client Rights

Counselors who offer distance counseling services and/or maintain a professional website provide electronic links to relevant licensure and professional certification boards to protect consumer and client rights and address ethical concerns.

H.5.c. Electronic Links

Counselors regularly ensure that electronic links are working and are professionally appropriate.

H.5.d. Multicultural and Disability Considerations

Counselors who maintain websites provide accessibility to persons with disabilities. They provide translation capabilities for clients who have a different primary language, when feasible. Counselors acknowledge the imperfect nature of such translations and accessibilities.

H.6. Social Media

H.6.a. Virtual Professional Presence

In cases where counselors wish to maintain a professional and personal presence for social media use, separate professional and personal web pages and profiles are created to clearly distinguish between the two kinds of virtual presence.

H.6.b. Social Media as Part of Informed Consent

Counselors clearly explain to their clients, as part of the informed consent procedure, the benefits, limitations, and boundaries of the use of social media.

H.6.c. Client Virtual Presence

Counselors respect the privacy of their clients' presence on social media unless given consent to view such information.

H.6.d. Use of Public Social Media

Counselors take precautions to avoid disclosing confidential information through public social media.

National Board for Certified Counselors (NBCC) Code of Ethics (2023)

TELEMENTAL HEALTH, SOCIAL MEDIA, AND TECHNOLOGY

Telemental Health

91. Counselors shall provide only those telemental health services for which they are qualified by education and experience.

92. Counselors shall carefully adhere to legal requirements when providing telemental health services. This requirement includes legal regulations from the State(s) in which the counselor and client are located. Counselors shall document relevant State requirements in the relevant client record(s).

93. Counselors shall ensure that the electronic means used in providing telemental health services are in compliance with current Federal and State laws and regulatory standards concerning telemental health service.

94. Counselors shall ensure that all electronic technology communications with clients are

encrypted and secure.

95. Counselors shall maintain records of all clinical contacts with telemental health service clients.

96. Counselors shall set clear expectations and boundaries with telemental health service recipients about the type(s) and timing of communications that will be included in service provision. These expectations and boundaries shall be communicated in writing in disclosure documents provided to clients.

97. Counselors shall provide written information to all telemental health clients regarding the protection of client records, accounts and related passwords, electronic communications, and client identity. This information should include a description of the nature of all communication security measures that are used by the counselor, including any risks or limitations related to the provision of telemental health services.

98. Counselors shall communicate information regarding security to clients who receive telemental health services. Telemental health service clients shall be informed of the potential risks of telemental health communications, including warnings about transmitting private information when using a public access computer or one that is on a shared network.

99. Counselors shall screen potential telemental health service clients to determine whether such services are appropriate. These considerations shall be documented in the client's record. Counselors shall advise telemental health services clients that they must be intentional about protecting their privacy and confidentiality, including advice concerning viewing employer policies relating to the possible prohibitions concerning the use of work computer systems for personal communications, and not using "auto-remember" usernames and passwords.

100. During the screening or intake process, Counselors shall provide potential clients with a detailed written description of the telemental health counseling process and service provision. This information shall be specific to the identified service delivery type, and include relevant considerations for that particular client. These considerations shall include: the appropriateness of telemental health counseling in relation to the specific goal; the format of service delivery; the electronic equipment requirements such as the need for a computer with certain capabilities; the limitations of confidentiality; privacy concerns; the possibility of technological failure; anticipated response time to electronic communication; alternate service delivery processes; and, any additional considerations necessary to assist the potential client in reaching a determination about the appropriateness of the telemental health service delivery format for their needs. Counselors shall discuss this information throughout the service delivery process to ensure that this method satisfies the anticipated goals. The counselor will document such information and the discussion of alternative service options and referrals in the client's record.

101. Counselors shall prevent the distribution of confidential telemental health client information to unauthorized individuals. Counselors shall

discuss actions the client may take to reduce the possibility that such confidential information is sent to unauthorized individuals in error.

102. Counselors shall provide clients of telemental health services with information concerning their professional preparation and/or credentials related to telemental health, and identify the relevant credentialing organization websites.

103. Counselors, either prior to or during the initial session, shall inform clients of the purposes, goals, procedures, limitations, and potential risks and benefits of telemental health services and techniques. Counselors also shall provide information about rights and responsibilities as appropriate to the telemental health service. Counselors also shall discuss with clients the associated challenges that may occur when communicating through telemental health means, including those associated with privacy and confidentiality.

104. In the event that the client of telemental health services is a minor or is unable to provide legal consent, the counselor shall obtain a legal guardian's consent prior to the provision of services unless otherwise required by State law. Counselors shall retain documentation indicating the legal guardian's identity and consent in the client's file.

105. Counselors will provide clients of telemental health services with specific written procedures regarding emergency assistance situations related to a client. This information shall include the identification of emergency responders near the client's location. Counselors shall take reasonable steps to secure referrals for recipients when needed for emergencies. Counselors shall provide information to clients concerning the importance of identifying personal contacts in the event of identified emergency situations, and shall ask clients to identify such contacts. Counselors also shall identify to the clients the circumstances in which the counselor will communicate with emergency contacts, and the information that will be shared with emergency contacts.

106. Counselors shall develop written procedures for verifying the identity of each telemental health client, their current location, and readiness to proceed at the beginning of each contact. Examples of verification include the use of code words, phrases, or inquiries, such as "Is this a good time to proceed?"

107. Counselors shall limit use of client information obtained through social media sources (e.g., Facebook, LinkedIn, Twitter) in accordance with established practice procedures provided to the client at the initiation of services and as adopted through the ongoing informed consent process.

108. Counselors shall retain telemental health service records for a minimum of five (5) years unless applicable State laws require additional time. Counselors shall limit the use of such client records to those permitted by

law and professional standards, and as specified by the agreement terms with the respective telemental health services client.

Social Media and Technology

109. Counselors shall provide services pursuant to an appropriate written policy which regulates the use of social media and other related digital technology with respect to current and former clients. This policy shall include terms that protect against the disclosure of confidential client information and the creation of multiple relationships. This policy shall also identify that client and counselor personal accounts are distinct from social media accounts used for professional purposes.
110. Counselors shall be familiar with the use of privacy and security settings of social media and other electronic platforms utilized for telemental health service provision. Counselors shall understand the purpose of those settings and their impact on client confidentiality, and ensure that such settings are in use.

111. Counselors shall not publish confidential client information on any social media platform, including updates, and blogs, without the consent of the client. To facilitate the secure provision of information, counselors shall inform clients prior to or during the initial session about secure and appropriate ways to communicate with them. Counselors also shall advise clients about the potential risks of sending messages through digital technology and social media sources.

112. Counselors who use digital technology for professional purposes shall only post information related to professional services, such as information concerning advocacy, educational purposes, and marketing, that does not create multiple relationships or threaten client confidentially.

113. Counselors shall respect the privacy of a client's social media material and accounts, and shall not access client social media accounts without specific client permission, a related discussion with the client, documentation of potential risks and benefits, and a specific clinical purpose.

114. Counselors shall avoid non-professional relationships with clients online. This restriction includes connecting with or following client social media accounts

References

Abdallah Altarawneh, A. M., & Awwad Alomoush, R. A. (2022). The reality of E-counseling services in the light of digital learning from the point of view of teachers in Jordan. *Education and Information Technologies, 27*(9), 12773–12792. https://doi.org/10.1007/s10639-022-11102-8

Acierno, R., Gros, D. F., Ruggiero, K. J., Hernandez-Tejada, B. M. A., Knapp, R. G., Lejuez, C. W., Muzzy, W., Frueh, C. B., Egede, L. E., & Tuerk, P. W. (2016). Behavioral activation and therapeutic exposure for post-traumatic stress disorder: A noninferiority trial of treatment delivered in person versus home-based telehealth. *Depression and Anxiety, 33*(5), 415–423. https://doi.org/10.1002/da.22476

Albalat Peraita, B. (2023, November 20). IAmorosexuality: a new sexual orientation? *The Conversation.* https://theconversation.com/iamorosexualidad-estamos-ante-una-nueva-orientacion-sexual-216368

Al-Halalmeh, S., & Al-Halalmeh, S. (2021). School counseling skills needed to activate distance learning in light of COVID-19 pandemic. *Turkish Journal of Computer and Mathematics Education, 12*(6), 1189–1194.

Alicata, D., Schropher, A., Unten, T., Aghora, R., Helm, S., Fukada, M., Ulrich, C., & Michaels, S. (2016). Telemental health training, team building, and workforce development in cultural contexts: The Hawaii experience. *Journal of Child and Adolescent Psychopharmacology, 3,* 260–265. https://doi.org/10.1089/cap.2015.0036

Alvarado, H. A. (2021, December 29). Telemedicine services in substance use and mental health treatment facilities. *Substance Abuse and Mental Health Services Administration (SAMHSA), Center for Behavioral Health Statistics and Quality.* https://www.samhsa.gov/data/report/telemedicine-services

American Academy of Pediatrics. (2016). Media and young minds. *Pediatrics, 138*(5), 1–6. https://pediatrics.aappublications.org/content/pediatrics/138/5/e20162591.full.pdf

American Association of Marriage and Family Therapy (AAMFT). (2015). *Code of ethics*. Author. https://www.aamft.org/Legal_Ethics/Code_of_Ethics.aspx

American Association for Marriage and Family Therapy Regulatory Boards. (2016). *Teletherapy guidelines*. https://amftrb.org/wp-content/uploa ds/2017/05/Proposed-Teletherapy-Guidelines-DRAFT-as-of-09.12.16.pdf

American Association of Sexuality Educators, Counselors, and Therapists (AASECT). (2020). *Code of conduct*. https://www.aasect.org/sites/default/files/documents/AASECT_Code-of-conduct-11.2020_4.20.23-edit_0.pdf

American Counseling Association. (2014). *Code of ethics*. https://www.counseling.org/knowledge-center/ethics

American Educational Research Association (AERA), American Psychological Association (APA), & National Council on Measurement in Education. (2014; 2024). *Standards for education and psychological testing*. AERA. https://www.testingstandards.net/open-access-files.html

American Mental Health Counselors Association. (2023). *AMHCA standards of practice of clinical mental health counseling*. https://www.amhca.org/viewdocument/2023-amhca-standards-for-the-practi

American Mental Health Counselors Association. (2020). *Code of ethics*. https://www.amhca.org/events/publications/ethics

American Psychiatric Association. (2021, May 27). *New nationwide poll shows an increased popularity for telehealth services*. https://psychiatry.org/news-room/news-releases/new-nationwide-poll-shows-an-increased-popularity

American Psychiatric Association. (2022). Desk reference to the diagnostic criteria from DSM-5-TR.

American Psychiatric Association. (2024). *App advisor: The app evaluation model*. https://www.psychiatry.org/psychiatrists/practice/mental-health-apps/the-app-evaluation-model

American School Counselors Association. (2022). *ASCA ethical standards for school counselors*. https://www.schoolcounselor.org/About-School-Counseling/Ethical-Legal-Responsibilities/ASCA-Ethical-Standards-for-School-Counselors-(1)

American Society of Addiction Medicine (ASAM). (2022). *ASAM Criteria Assessment Interview*. Author.

Anthony, K. (2015). Training therapists to work effectively online and offline within digital culture. *British Journal of Guidance & Counselling, 43*(1), 36–42, http://doi.org/10.1080/03069885.2014.924617

Arizona State University. (2023, August 14). ASU projects record enrollment for fall 2023. https://news.asu.edu/20230814-sun-devil-life-asu-projects-record-enrollment-fall-2023

Arnberg, F. K., Linton, S. J., Hultcrantz, M., Heintz, E., & Jonsson, U. (2014). Internet-delivered psychological treatments for mood and anxiety disorders: A systematic review of their efficacy, safety, and cost-effectiveness. *PLOS ONE, 9*(5), e98118. https://doi.org/10.1371/journal.pone.0098118

Assistive Technology Industry Association (ATIA). (2024). https://www.atia.org/

Association for Specialists in Group Work. (2021) *Guiding principles for group work.* https://asgw.org/wp-content/uploads/2021/07/ASGW-Guiding-Principles-May-2021.pdf

Astin, A. W. (1984). Student involvement: A developmental theory for higher education. *Journal of College Student Personnel, 25*(4), 297–308.

Auxier, B., & Anderson, M. (2021, April 16). Social media use in 2021. https://www.pewresearch.org/internet/2021/04/07/social-media-use-in-2021/

Avent Harris, J. R., Crumb, L., Crowe, A., & Garland McKinney, J. (2020). African Americans' perceptions of mental illness and preferences for treatment. *Journal of Counselor Practice, 11*(1), 1–22. https://doi.org/10.22229/afa1112020

Baber, T. F., Higgins-Biddle, J. C., Saunders, J. B., & Monteiro, M. G. (2001). *Alcohol Use Disorders Identification Test (AUDIT)* (2nd ed.). World Health Organization (WHO).

Baird, M. B., Whitney, L., & Caedo, C. E. (2018). Experiences and attitudes among psychiatric mental health advanced practice nurses in the use of telemental health: Results of an online survey. *Journal of the American Psychiatric Nurses Association, 24*(3) 235–240. https://doi.org/10.1177/1078390317717330

Barker, G. G., & Barker, E. E. (2022). Online therapy: Lessons learned from the COVID-19 health crisis. *British Journal of Guidance & Counselling, 50*(1), 66–81.

Barker, M-J., & Iantaffi, A. (2019). *Life isn't binary: One being both, beyond, and in-between.* Jessica Kingsley Publishers.

Barrio, P., Ortega, L., Lopez, H., & Gual, A. (2017). Self-management and shared decision-making in alcohol dependence via mobile app: A pilot study. *International Journal of Behavioral Medicine, 24,* 722–727. https://doi.org/10.1007/s12529-017-9643-6

Bitondo Dyer, C., Murdock, C., Hiner, J., Halphen, J., & Burnett, J. (2020). Elder mistreatment intervention: Strategies for connecting with diverse and rural populations. *Journal of the American Society on Aging, 44*(1), 91–97. https://www.jstor.org/stable/26992874

Blumer, M., Hertlein, K. M., & VanderBosch, M. (2015). Towards the development of educational core competencies for couple and family therapy technology practices. *Contemporary Family Therapy, 37,* 113–121.https://doi.org/10.1007/s1059 1-015-9330-1

Boniel-Nissim, M. (2016). Using forums to enhance client peer support. In S. Goss, K. Anthony, L. Sykes Stretch, & Merz Nagel, D. (Eds.) *Technology in mental health: Applications in practice, supervision, and training.* Charles C. Thomas Publishers.

Borenstein, L. (2022). Imagination and play in teletherapy with children. *American Journal of Play, 14,* 13–32. https://doi.org/10.1111/ajad.12805

Breen, G. M., & Matusitz, J. (2010). An evolutionary examination of telemedicine: A health and computer-mediated communication perspective. *Social Work Public Health, 25*(1): 59–71. https://doi.org/10.1080/19371910902911206

Brott, P. E., & Willis, D. A. (2021). Vlogging as a tool in the self-reflective journey: Professional identity development as a space between. *Sage Open, 11*(4). https://doi.org/10.1177/21582440211061526

Brown, D. (2016). *Career information, career counseling, and career development* (11th ed.). Pearson.

Cameron, S., & Turtle-Song, I. (2002). Learning to write case notes using the SOAP format. *Journal of Counseling & Development, 80,* 286–292.

Cantor, J., McBain, R. K., Kofner, A., Hanson, R., Stein, B. D., & Yu, H. (2021). Telehealth adoption by mental health and substance use disorder treatment facilities in the COVID-19 pandemic. *Psychiatric Services, 73,* 365–477. https://doi.org/10.1176/appi.ps.202100191

Carlbring, P., Degerman, N., Jonsson, J., & Andersson, G. (2012). Internet-based treatment of pathological gambling with a three-year follow-up. *Cognitive Behaviour Therapy, 41*(4), 321–335. https://doi.org/10.1080/16506073.2012.689323

Carpenter, A. L., Pincus, D. B., Furr, J. M., & Comer, J. S. (2018). Working from home: An initial pilot examination of videoconferencing-based cognitive behavioral therapy for anxious youth delivered to the home setting. *Behaivor Therapy, 49,* 917–930. https://doi.org/10.1016/j.beth.2018.01.007

Celio, M. A., Mastroleo, N. R., DiGuiseppi, G., Barnett, N. P., Colby, S. M., Kahler, C. W., ... Monti, P. M. (2017). Using video conferencing to deliver brief motivational intervention for alcohol and sex risk to emergency department patients: A proof-of-concept pilot study. *Addiction Research & Theory, 25,* 318–325. http://doi.org/10.1080/16066359.2016.1276902

Center for Credentialing in Education (CCE). (2024). *BC-TMH: Board certified telemental health provider.* https://www.cce-global.org/credentialing/bctmh

Center for Connected Health Policy. (n.d.). *What is telehealth?* https://www.cchpca.org/what-is-telehealth/

Centers for Disease Control and Prevention. (2020). *Telehealth and telemedicine.* https://www.cdc.gov/phlp/publications/topic/telehealth.html

Centers for Medicaid and Medicare Services. (n.d.). *Telemedicine.* https://www.medicaid.gov/medicaid/benefits/telemedicine/index.html

Chen, S.-Y., Coker, K., Wathen, C., & Sheperis, D. (2021) Effects of clinical skills training: Technology and pedagogy for the quality virtual classroom. *Journal of Technology in Counselor Education and Supervision, 1,* 9. https://digital.sandiego.edu/tces/vol1/iss1/9

Chickering A. W. & Reisser, L. (1993). *Education and identity* (2nd ed.) Jossey-Bass.

Choi, D. S., Park, J., Loeser, M. & Seo, K. (2024). Improving counseling effectiveness with virtual counselors through nonverbal compassion involving eye contact, facial mimicry, and head-nodding. *Sci Rep, 14,* 506. https://doi.org/10.1038/s41598-023-51115-y

Choudhuri, D. D. (2020). Working virtually in group work. https://asgw.org/resources/#tab-virtualgroups

Cipoletta, S., & Mocellin, D. (2018). Online counseling: An exploratory survey of Italian psychologists' attitudes toward new ways of interaction. *Psychotherapy Research, 28,* 909–924. https://doi.org/10.1080/10503307.2016.1259533

Coker, K., Snow, W., & Hinkle, S. (2021). The past, present, and future of online counselor education. *Journal of Technology in Counselor Education and Supervision, 1*(1), 6. https://digital.sandiego.edu/tces/vol1/iss1/6/

Colbow, A. J. (2013). Looking to the future: Integrating telemental health therapy into psychologist training. *Training and Education in Professional Psychology, 3*(2), 155–165. https://doi.org/10.1037/a0033454

Comer, J. S., Furr, J. M., Miguel, E. M., Cooper-Vince, C. E., Carpenter, A. L., Elkins, R. M., ... Chase, R. (2017). Remotely delivering real-time parent training in the home: An initial randomized trial of internet-delivered Parent-Child Interaction Therapy (I-PCIT). *Journal of Consulting and Clinical Psychology, 85*(9), 909–917. http://dx.doi.org/10.1037/ccp0000230

Commission on Rehabilitation Counselor Certification. (2023). *Code of professional ethics for Certified Rehabilitation Counselors.* https://crccertification.com/code-of-ethics-4/

Community Technical Assistance Center of New York (CTACNY). (2020, April). *Telemental Health Tip Sheets: Virtual group therapy.* https://www.ctacny.org/series/

Conners, C. K. (2022). *Conners 4th Edition.* Pearson.

Corey, D. M., & Ben-Porath, Y. S. (2020). Practical guidance on the use of the MMPI instruments in remote psychological testing. *Professional Psychology: Research and Practice, 51*(3), 199–204. http://doi.org/10.1037/pro0000329

Council on the Accreditation of Counseling and Related Education Programs. (2023). *CACREP standards.* https://www.cacrep.org/for-programs/

Council for the Advancement of Standards (CAS) in Higher Education. (2023). *Standards.* Author. https://www.cas.edu/standards.html

Counseling Compact. (2024). https://counselingcompact.org/

Courage, M. L., Bakhtiar, A., Fitzpatrick, C., Kenny, S., & Brandeau, K. (2015). Growing up multitasking: The costs and benefits for cognitive development. *Developmental Review, 35,* 5–41. http://doi.org/10.1016/j.dr.2014.12.002

Creed, T. A., Kuo, P. B., Oziel, R., Reich, D., Thomas, M., O'Connor, S., Imel, Z. E., Hirsch, T., Narayanan, S., & Atkins, D. C. (2022). Knowledge and attitudes toward an artificial intelligence-based fidelity measurement in community cognitive behavioral therapy supervision. *Administration and Policy in Mental Health, 49,* 343–356. https://doi.org/10.1007/s10488-021-01167-x

Cruz, B. N., Miller, E., & Chen, R. K. (2022). Social media use and depression among young adults: Rehabilitation counseling implications. *Journal of Applied Rehabilitation Counseling, 53*(3), 228–243. https://doi.org/10.1891/JARC-D-21-00002

Donovan, D. (2024). Exploring the role of social media use in eating disorders in adolescents: A scoping review. *Mental Health Practice, 27*(3), 31–36. https://doi.org/10.7748/mhp.2024.e1690

Dorstyn, D., Oxlad, M., Roberts, R., Murphy, G., Potter, E., Kneebone, I., & Craig, A. (2022). MS JobSeek: A pilot randomized controlled trial of an online peer discussion forum for job-seekers with multiple sclerosis. *Journal of Vocational Rehabilitation, 56*(1), 81–91. https://doi.org/10.3233/JVR-211174

Epstein, Becker, Green. (2024). *Telemental Health Laws App.* https://www.ebglaw.com/telemental-health-laws-app

Epstein, J., & Bequette, A. W. (2013). Smart phone applications in clinical practice. *Journal of Mental Health Counseling, 35*(4), 283–295. https://doi.org/10.17744/mehc.35.4.f85k258620765tj4

Evans, K. M., & Sejuit, A. L. (2021). *Gaining cultural competence in career counseling* (2nd ed.). National Career Development Association.

Forsell, E., Bendix, M., Holländare, F., Szymanska von Schultz, B., Nasiell, J., Blomdahl-Wetterholm, M., Eriksson, C., Kvarned, S., Lindau van der Linden, J., Söderberg, E., Jokinen, J., Wide, K., & Kaldo, V. (2017). Internet-delivered cognitive behavior therapy for antenatal depression: A randomised controlled trial. *Journal of Affective Disorders, 221,* 56–64. https://doi.org/10.1016/j.jad.2017.06.013

Freed. (2023a). How Freed works. https://www.home.getfreed.ai/

Freed. (2023b). Freed Privacy and Security. https://www.home.getfreed.ai/privacy-policy

Froehlich, R. J., Henry, J. S., Tichy, N., Hill, J. C., & Thompson, K. (2023). Rehabilitation counselors and technology, social media, and distance counseling: Contemporary considerations. *Rehabilitation Counseling Bulletin, 66*(4), 265–273. https://doi.org/10.1177/00343552221147219

Ghosh, S. (2020, November 2). NUIA Full Focus launched as a smart software for natural eye contact in video calls. *AiTHORITY: AI Technology Insights.* https://aithority.com/vision/

video-understanding/nuia-full-focus-launched-as-a-smart-software-for-natural-eye-contact-in-video-calls/

Gilbertson, J. (2020). *Telemental health: The essential guide to providing successful online therapy.* PESI Publishing & Media.

Glover, J. A., Williams, E., Hazlett, L. J., & Campbell, N. (2013). Connecting to the future: Telepsychiatry in post graduate medical education. *Telemedicine and e-Health, 19*(6), 474–479. https://doi.org/10.1089/tmj.2012.0182

Globokar, R. (2018). Impact of digital media on emotional, social, and moral development. *Nova Prisutnost, 3,* 545–560.

Gluek, D. (2013). Establishing therapeutic rapport in telemental health. In Myers, K., & Turvey, C. L. (Eds.), *Telemental health: Clinical and administrative foundations for evidence-based practice* (pp. 65–82). Elsevier.

Gonzales, G., de Mola, E. L., Robertson, L., Gavulic, K. A., & McKay, T. (2023). LGBTQ college student health and wellbeing at the onset of the pandemic: Additional evidence and lessons learned from COVID-19. *BMC Public Health, 23*(1), Article 15909. https://doi.org/10.1186/s12889-023-15909-z

Goss, S., Anthony, K., Stretch, L.S., & Nagel, D. M. (2016). *Technology in mental health: Applications in practice, supervision, and training.* Charles C. Thomas.

Goss, S., & Ferns, J. (2016). Using cell/mobile phone SMS to enhance client crisis and peer support. In Goss, S., Anthony, K., Stretch, L.S., & Nagel, D. M. (Eds.). *Technology in mental health: Applications in practice, supervision, and training* (pp. 123–140). Charles C. Thomas.

Grondin, F., Lomanowska, A. M., Poiré, V., & Jackson, P. L. (2022). Clients in simulated teletherapy via videoconference compensate for altered eye contact when evaluating therapist empathy. *Journal of Clinical Medicine, 11*(12), Article 3461. https://doi.org/10.3390/jcm11123461

Grondin, F., Lomanowska, A. M., Békés V., & Jackson, P. L. (2021) A methodology to improve eye contact in telepsychotherapy via videoconferencing with considerations for psychological distance. *Counselling Psychology Quarterly, 34*(4), 586–599, https://doi.org/10.1080/09515070.2020.1781596

Guth, L. J., Pepper, E. L., & Garrow, J. (2020). Ten tips for the facilitation of virtual groups. *ASGW Resources.* https://asgw.org/resources/#tab-virtualgroups

Haberstroh, S., Parr, G., Bradley, L., Morgan-Flemming, B., & Gee, R. (2008). Facilitating online counseling: Perspectives from counselors in training. *Journal of Counseling & Development, 86*(4), 460–470. https://doi.org/10.1002/j.1556-6678.2008.tb00534.x

Haeger, J. A., Davis, C. H., & Levin, M. E. (2022). Utilizing ACT daily as a self-guided app for clients waiting for services at a college counseling center: A pilot study. *Journal of American College Health, 70*(7), 742–749. https://doi.org/10.1080/07448481.2020.1763366

Han, M., & Pong, H. (2015). Mental health help-seeking behaviors among Asian American community college students: The effect of stigma, cultural barriers, and acculturation. *Journal of College Student Development 56*(1), 1–14. https://doi.org/10.1353/csd.2015.0001.

Hargittai, E., & Dobransky, K. (2017). Old dogs, new clicks: Digital inequality in skills and uses among older adults. *Canadian Journal of Communication, 42*(2), 195–212. http://doi.org/10.22230/cjc2017v42n2a3176

Harris-Bowlsbey, J., & Sampson, J. P. (2005). Use of technology in delivering career services worldwide. *The Career Development Quarterly, 54*(1), 48–56. https://doi.org/10.1002/j.2161-0045.2005.tb00143.x

Health Resources and Services Administration. (2019, August 16). *Shortage areas. HRSA*. https://data.hrsa.gov/topics/health-workforce/shortage-areas

Hertlein, K. M., Drude, K. P., Hilty, D. M., & Maheu, M. M. (2021). Toward proficiency in telebehavioral health: applying interprofessional competencies in couple and family therapy. *Journal of Marital and Family Therapy, 47*(2), 359–374. https://doi.org/10.1111/jmft.12496

Hertlein, K. M., & Twist, M. L. C. (2019). *The internet family: Technology in couple and family relationships.* Routledge.

Hilty, D. M., Crawford, A., Teshima, J., Chan, S., Sunderji, N., Yellowlees, P. M., Kramer, G., O'Neill, P., Fore, C., Luo, J., & Li, S. (2015). A framework for telepsychiatric training and e-health: Competency-based education, evaluation and implications. *International Review of Psychiatry, 27*(6), 569–592. http://doi.org/10.3109/09540261.2015.1091292

Hobbs, M. J., Joubert, A. E., Mahoney, A. E. J., & Andrews, G. (2018). Treating late-life depression: Comparing the effects of internet-delivered cognitive behavior therapy across the lifespan. *Journal of Affective Disorders, 226,* 58–65. https://doi.org/10.1016/j.jad.2017.10.013

Hoffman, P., & Kane, J. M. (2013). Telepsychiatry education and curriculum development in residency training. *Academic Psychiatry, 39*(2), 108–109. https://doi.org/10.1007/s40596-013-0006-6

Hofstra University (n.d.). Saltzman Center Phobia and Trauma Clinic. https://www.hofstra.edu/saltzman-center/phobia-trauma-clinic.html

Holmes, C. M., & Reid, C. A. (2018). Ethics in telerehabilitation: Looking ahead. *Journal of Applied Rehabilitation Counseling, 49*(2), 14–23. https://doi.org/10.1891/0047-2220.49.2.14

Hooley, T., & Dodd, V. (2016). Online research methods for mental health. In S. Goss, K. Anthony, L. Sykes Stretch, & D. M. Nagel (Eds.), *Technology in mental health: Applications in practice, supervision, and training* (pp. 45–63). Charles C. Thomas Publishers.

Hornblow, A. R. (1986). The evolution and effectiveness of telephone counseling services. *Hospital and Community Psychiatry, 37*(8), 731–733.

Hornor, T., & Westberry, L. A. (2023). Virtual school counselling and COVID-19 as seen through an organizational learning lens. *International Journal of Education Policy and Leadership, 19*(1). https://doi.org/10.22230/ijepl.2023.19.1.1036

Human Resources Services Administration (HRSA). (2022, March). *What is telehealth?* https://www.hrsa.gov/rural-health/topics/telehealth/what-is-telehealth

Human Resources Services Administration (HRSA). (2023, January). *Health Workforce Shortage Areas.* https://data.hrsa.gov/topics/health-workforce/shortage-areas

Hunter, D., & Rewa, J. (2020). *Leading groups online: A down and dirty guide to leading online courses, meetings, trainings, and events during the coronavirus pandemic.* Authors.

Huskamp, H. A., Busch, A. B., Souza, J., Uscher-Pines, L., Rose, S., Wilcock, A., ... Mehrotra, A. (2018). How is telemedicine being used in opioid and other substance use disorder treatment? *Health Affairs, 37*(12), 1940–1947. https://doi.org/10.1377/hlthaff.2018.05134

IAmorosexuality: a new sexual orientation? (2024, January 3). *CE Noticias Financieras.* https://www.proquest.com/wire-feeds/iamorosexuality-new-sexual-orientation/docview/2910108510/se-2

Inman, A. G., Bashian, H., Pendse, A. C., & Luu, L. P. (2019). Publication trends in telesupervision: A content analysis study. *The Clinical Supervisor, 38*(1), 97–115. https://doi.org/10.1080/07325223.2018.1528194

International Association of Marriage and Family Counselors. (2017). *Code of ethics*. Author. https://www.iamfconline.org/public/department3.cfm

Jaconis, M., Santa Ana, E., Killeen, T. K., Badour, C. L., & Back, S. E. (2017). Concurrent treatment of PTSD and alcohol use disorder via telehealth in a female Iraq veteran: A case series. *The American Journal on Addictions, 26*(2), 112–114. https://doi.org/10.1111/ajad.12481

Johnson, D. (2021, March 15). What is a digital footprint? How to protect yourself online and keep your data from being used against you. *Business Insider.* https://www.businessinsider.com/guides/tech/what-is-a-digital-footprint

Jones, M. K., Leath, S., Latimer, K., Lawson, E., & Briones, M. (2022). The impact of COVID-19 on Black college students' mental health. *Journal of College Student Development, 63*(3), 239–254. https://doi.org/10.1353/csd.2022.0021

Kister, K., Laskowski, J., Makarewicz, A., & Tarkowski, J. (2023). Application of artificial intelligence tools in diagnosis and treatment of mental disorders. *Current Problems of Psychiatry, 24*(1), 1–18. https://doi.org/10.12923/2353-8627/2023-0001

Knowles, M. S. (1975). Adult education: New dimensions. *Educational Leadership, 33*(2), 85–91.

Knowles, K. (2017). What the heck is... teledildonics? *Forbes.* https://www.forbes.com/sites/kittyknowles/2017/02/09/teledildonics-meaning-what-are-teledildonics-iot-sex-toys-vr-porn/?sh=48473e755565

Kozlowski, K. A., & Holmes, C. M. (2014). Experiences in online process groups: A qualitative study. *Journal for Specialists in Group Work, 39*(3), 276–300. https://doi.org/10.1080/01933922.2014.948235

Kozlowski, K. A., & Holmes, C. M. (2017). Teaching online group counseling skills in an on-campus group counseling course. *The Journal of Counselor Preparation and Supervision, 9*(1), Article 6. https://doi.org/10.7729/91.1157

Krach, S. K., Paskiewicz, T. L., & Monk, M. M. (2020). Testing our children when the world shuts down: Analyzing recommendations for adapted tele-assessment during COVID-19. *Journal of Psychoeducational Assessment, 38*(8), 923–941. https://doi.org/10.1177/0734282920962839

Kus, M., & Aydin, M. K. (2022). Teachers' views on guidance and counseling services at schools during the COVID-19 pandemic: Challenges and opportunities. *Education Quarterly Reviews, 5*(3), 9–18.

Larson, L. M., Suzuki, L. A., Gillespie, K. N., Potenza, M. T., Bechtel, M. A., & Toulouse, A. L. (1992). Development and validation of the Counseling Self-Estimate Inventory. *Journal of Counseling Psychology, 39*(1), 105–120. https://doi.org/10.1037/0022-0167.39.1.105

Lawes-Wickwar, S., McBain, H., & Mulligan, K. (2018). Application and effectiveness of telehealth to support severe mental illness management: Systematic review. *JMIR Ment Health 5*(4), Article e62. https://doi.org/10.2196/mental.8816

Lent, R. W., Hill, C. E., & Hoffman, M. A. (2003). Development and validation of the Counselor Activity Self-Efficacy Scales. *Journal of Counseling Psychology, 50,* 97–108. https://psycnet.apa.org/doi/10.1037/0022-0167.50.1.97

Lütt, A., Tsamitros, N., Wolbers, T., Rosenthal, A., Bröcker, A. L., Schöneck, R., Bermpohl, F., Heinz, A., Beck, A., & Gutwinski, S. (2023). An explorative single-arm clinical study to assess craving in patients with alcohol use disorder using virtual reality exposure (CRAVE)—Study protocol. *BMC Psychiatry, 23*(1), Article 53. https://doi.org/10.1186/s12888-023-05346-y

Lutxon, D. D., Nelson, E., & Maheu, M. M. (2023). A practitioner's guide to telemental health: *How to conduct legal, ethical, and evidence-based telepractice* (2nd ed.). American Psychological Association.

Marr, B. (2023, May 19). A short history of ChatGPT and how we got here. *Forbes.* https://www.forbes.com/sites/bernardmarr/2023/05/19/a-short-history-of-chatgpt-how-we-got-to-where-we-are-today/?sh=69c4994e674f

Matheu, M. (2017). *Career paths in telemental health.* Springer.

Malone, J. F., Miller, R. K., & Walz, G. R. (Eds.). (2007). *Distance counseling: Expanding the counselor's reach and impact.* Counseling Outfitters.

Mariani, M. (1999, Spring). Replace with a database: O*NET replaces the Dictionary of Occupational Titles. *Occupational Outlook Quarterly.* https://www.bls.gov/careeroutlook/1999/Spring/art01.pdf

Martin, P., Lizarondo, L., & Kumar, S. (2018). A systematic review of the factors that influence the quality and effectiveness of telesupervision for health professionals. *Journal of Telemedicine and Telecare, 24*(4), 271–281. https://doi.org/10.1177/1357633X17698868

Mark, T. L., Treiman, K., Padwa, H., Henretty, K., Tzeng, J., & Gilbert, M. (2021). Addiction treatment and telehealth: Review of efficacy and provider insights during the COVID-19 pandemic. *Psychiatric Services, 73*(5), 481–491. https://doi.org/10.1176/appi.ps.202100088

Masho, S. W., & Alvanzo, A. (2010). Help-seeking behavior among men sexual assault survivors. *American Journal of Men's Health, 4*(3), 237–242. https://doi.org/10.1177/1557988309336365

McArthur, N., & Twist, M. L. C. (2017). The rise of digisexuality: therapeutic challenges and possibilities. *Sexual and Relationship Therapy, 32*(3–4), 334–344. https://doi.org/10.1080/14681994.2017.1397950

McCarty, C. A., Vander Stoep, A., Violette, H., & Myers, K. (2015). Interventions developed for psychiatric and behavioral treatment in the children's ADHD telemental health treatment study. *Journal of Child and Family Studies, 24*(6), 1735–1743. https://doi.org/10.1007/s10826-014-9977-5

McLean, S. A., Booth, A. T., Schnabel, A., Wright, B. J., Painter, F. L., & McIntosh, J. E. (2021). Exploring the efficacy of telehealth for family therapy through systematic, meta-analytic, and qualitative evidence. *Clinical Child and Family Psychology Review, 24*(2), 244–266. https://doi.org/10.1007/s10567-020-00340-2

Medalia, A., Lynch, D. A., & Herlands, T. (2020). Telehealth conversion of serious mental illness recovery services during the COVID-19 crisis. *Psychiatric Services, 71*(8), 872–873. https://doi.org/10.1176/appi.ps.71705

Medina Greenspan, H., Broadbent, M., Zhang, X., Axford, K. E., Kious, B., Imel, Z., & Srikumar, V. (2023, July 9–14). Logic-driven indirect supervision: An application in crisis counseling [Paper presentation]. *Association for Computational Linguistics 61st Annual Meeting*. https://aclanthology.org/2023.acl-long.654.pdf

Mehrotra, A., Huskamp, H. A., Souza, J., Uscher-Pines, L., Rose, S., Landon, B. E., ... Busch, A. B. (2017). Rapid growth in mental health telemedicine use among rural Medicare beneficiaries: Wide variation across states. *Health Affairs, 36*(5), 909–917. https://doi.org/10.1377/hlthaff.2016.1461

Menendez, J., Franco, M., Davari, J., Gnilka, P. B., & Ashby, J. S. (2020). Barriers and facilitators to Latinx college students seeking counseling. *Journal of College Student Psychotherapy, 34*(4), 302–315, https://doi.org/10.1080/87568225.2019.1600093

Miegel, F., Bücker, L., Kühn, S., Mostajeran, F., Moritz, S., Baumeister, A., Lohse, L., Blömer, J., Grzella, K., & Jelinek, L. (2022). Exposure and response prevention in virtual reality for patients with contamination-related obsessive–compulsive disorder: A case series. *Psychiatric Quarterly, 93*(3), 861–882. https://doi.org/10.1007/s11126-022-09992-5

Miu, A., S., Vo, H. T., Palka, J. M., Glowacki, C. R., & Robinson, R. J. (2021) Teletherapy with serious mental illness populations during COVID-19: telehealth conversion and engagement. *Counselling Psychology Quarterly, 34*(4), 704–721. https://doi.org/10.1080/09515070.2020.1791800

Molfenter, T., Brown, R., O'Neill, A., Kopetsky, E., & Toy, A. (2018). Use of telemedicine in addiction treatment: Current practices and organizational implementation characteristics. *International Journal of Telemedicine and Applications*, Article 3932643. https://doi.org/10.1155/2018/3932643

Molnar, A. (Ed.), Miron, G., Barbour, M. K., Huerta, L., Shafer, S. R., Rice, J. K., Glover, A., Browning, N., Hagle, S., & Boninger, F. (2021). *Virtual schools in the US 2021.* National Education Policy Center. http://nepc.colorado.edu/publication/virtual-schools-annual-2021

Moody, J. (2019, October 3). 10 schools with the most online students. *U.S. News and World Report*. https://www.usnews.com/higher-education/online-education/slideshows/schools-with-the-most-online-students

Morgen, K., Miller, G., & Stretch, L. S. (2012). Addiction counseling licensure issues for licensed professional counselors. *The Professional Counselor, 2*(1), 58–65.

Myers, K., & Turvey, C. L. (Eds.). (2013). *Telemental health: Clinical and administrative foundations for evidence-based practice.* Elsevier.

NAADAC: The Association for Addiction Professionals. (2021). *NAADAC/NCC AP code of ethics*. https://www.naadac.org/code-of-ethics

National Board for Certified Counselors. (1997). Standards for the ethical practice of WebCounseling, *NBCC News Notes, 14*(2), 3–4. http://www.nbcc.org/Assets/Newsletter/Issues/fall97.pdf

National Board for Certified Counselors. (2016). *Policy regarding the provision of distance professional services*. https://nbcc.org/ethics

National Board for Certified Counselors. (2023). *NBCC code of ethics.* https://nbcc.org/ethics

National Career Development Association. (2015). *Ethical use of social networking technologies in career services*. https://ncda.org/aws/NCDA/asset_manager/get_file/110167?ver=53186

National Career Development Association. (2024). *Code of ethics*. https://www.ncda.org/aws/NCDA/asset_manager/get_file/3395

National Institute of Mental Health. (2021). *Technology and the future of mental health treatment*. https://www.nimh.nih.gov/health/topics/technology-and-the-future-of-mental-health-treatment

National Institute of Mental Health. (n.d.). *What is telehealth?* https://www.nimh.nih.gov/health/publications/what-is-telemental-health

Neely-Fairbanks, S. Y., Rojas-Guyler, L., Nabors, L., & Banjo, O. (2018). Mental illness knowledge, stigma, help-seeking behaviors, spirituality, and the African American church. *American Journal of Health Studies, 33*(4), 162–174. http://www.va-ajhs.com/33-4/index.aspx

New York State Department of Education. (2020, April 6). *Board of Regents acts on series of emergency regulations to ease burdens of educators, students, and professionals in the wake of the COVID-19 pandemic*. https://www.nysed.gov/news/2023/board-regents-acts-series-emergency-regulations-ease-burdens-educators-students-and

Niles, S. G., Goodman, J., & Pope, M. (2013). *The career counseling casebook: A resource for students, practitioners, and counselor educators* (2nd ed.). National Career Development Association.

Osborn, D. S., Carr, D. L., McClain Riner, M., Sides, R. D., Lumsden, J. A., & Sampson, J. P. (2019). Computer-assisted career assessment. In K. B. Stoltz, & S. R. Barclay (Eds.). *A comprehensive guide to career assessment* (7th ed., pp. 321–335). National Career Development Association.

Ostrowski, J., & Collins, T. (2016). A comparison of telemental health terminology used across mental health state licensing boards. *The Professional Counselor, 6*(4) 387–396. https://doi.org/10.15241/jo.6.4.387

Paulino, R. A. (2022, September 15). Analyzing distance learning and flexible offerings during the COVID-19 era and the possible impact on future practices. *NASPA Student Affairs Administrators in Higher Education*. https://www.naspa.org/blog/analyzing-distance-learning-and-flexible-offerings-during-the-covid-19-era-and-the-possible-impact-on-future-practices

Pearson Inc. (2021). *Telepractice and questionnaires or rating scales*. https://www.pearsonassessments.com/professional-assessments/digital-solutions/telepractice/telepractice-and-the-mmpi-3.html

Parikh, S. B., Janson, C., & Singleton, T. (2012). Video journaling as a method of reflective practice. *Counselor Education and Supervision, 51*, 33–49. https://doi.org/10.1002/j.1556-6978.2012.00003.x

Patel, S. Y., Huskamp, H. A., Busch, A. B., & Mehrotra, A. (2020). Telemental health and US rural–urban differences in specialty mental health use, 2010–2017. *American Journal of Public Health, 110*(9), 1308–1314. https://doi.org/10.2105/AJPH.2020.305657

Pea, R., & Cole, M. (2019). The living hand of the past: The role of technology in development. *Human Development, 62*(1–2), 14–39. https://doi.org/10.1159/000496073

Pedersen, P. B. (1991). Multiculturalism as a generic approach to counseling. *Journal of Counseling & Development, 70*(1), 6–12. https://doi.org/10.1002/j.1556-6676.1991.tb01555.x

Penn State. (2023). *Social and behavioral research: Use of social media as a research activity*. https://irb.upenn.edu/homepage/social-behavioral-homepage/guidance/types-of-social-behavioral-research/use-of-social-media-as-a-research-activity/

Perle, J. G., Langsam, L. C., Randel, A., Lutchman, S., Levine, A. B., Odland, A. P., Nierenberg, B., & Marker, C. D. (2012). Attitudes toward psychological telehealth: Current and future clinical psychologists' opinions of internet-based interventions. *Journal of Clinical Psychology, 69*, 100–113. https://doi.org/10.1002/jclp.21912

Perrin, A. (2021, June 3). Mobile technology and home broadband. *Pew Research Center*. https://www.pewresearch.org/internet/2021/06/03/mobile-technology-and-home-broadband-2021/

Perry, W. G., Jr. (1968). *Forms of intellectual and ethical development in the college years: A scheme*. Holt, Rinehart, & Winston.

Pew Research Center. (2021, April 7). *Internet/Broadband Fact Sheet*. https://www.pewresearch.org/internet/fact-sheet/internet-broadband/

Phillips, M. L. (2011). Using social media in your research: Experts explore the practicalities of observing human behavior through Facebook and Twitter. *American Psychological Association, gradPsych, 11*. https://www.apa.org/gradpsych/2011/11/social-media

Pogoda, T. K., Keleher, V., Marchany, K., Zogas, A., Dillahunt-Aspillaga, C. J., Might, R., Yee, J., & Carlson, K. F. (2021). Implementing supported employment for veterans with traumatic brain injury through remote counseling during COVID-19. *Journal of Rehabilitation, 87*(1), 64–70.

Posner, K., Brown, G. K., Stanley, B., Brent, D. A., Yershova, K. V., Oquendo, M. A., Currier, G. W., Melvin, G. A., Greenhill, L., Shen, S., & Mann, J. J. The Columbia-Suicide Severity Rating Scale: Initial validity and internal consistency findings from three multisite studies with adolescents and adults. *Am J Psychiatry, 168*(12):1266–77. https://doi.org/10.1176/appi.ajp.2011.10111704

Predmore, Z., Ramchand, R., Ayer, L., Kotzias, V., Engel, C., Ebener, P., ... Hass, G. L. (2017). Expanding suicide crisis services to text and chat. *Crisis, 38*(4), 255–260. https://doi.org/10.1027/0227-5910/a000460

Prensky, M. (2001). *Digital natives, digital immigrants.* https://www.marcprensky.com/writing/Prensky%20-%20Digital%20Natives,%20Digital%20Immigrants%20-%20Part1.pdf

Pullen, S. J., White, J. C., Salgado, C. A., Sengupta, S., Takala, C. R., Tai, S., Swintak, C., & Shatkin, J. P. (2013). Video-teleconferencing with medical students to improve exposure to child and adolescent psychiatry. *Academic Psychiatry, 34*(4), 268–270. https://doi.org/10.1176/appi.ap.12040073

Raja, M., & Lakshmi Priya, G. G. (2021). Conceptual origins, technological advancements, and impacts of using virtual reality technology in education. *Webology, 18*(2). https://doi.org/10.14704/web/v18i2/web18311

Ratts, M. J. (2009). Social justice counseling: Toward the development of a fifth force in thecounseling paradigm. *Journal of Humanistic Education, Counseling, and Development, 48,* 160–172.

Ratts, M. J., Singh, A. A., Nassar-McMillan, S., Butler, S. K., & Rafferty McCullough, J. (2015). *Multicultural and Social Justice Counseling Competencies.* https://www.counseling.org/docs/default-source/competencies/multicultural-and-social-justice-counseling-competencies.pdf

Rehabilitation Engineering and Assistive Technology Society of North America (RESNA). (2024). https://www.resna.org/

Robertson, H. (2013). Common crisis. *ASCA School Counselor,* March/April 2013, 41–45.

Robertson, H. C. (2021). *Telemental health and distance counseling: A counselor's guide to decisions, resources, and practice.* Springer Publishing Company.

Robertson, H. C., & Lowell, R. (2021). Counselor educator, supervisor, and practitioner perceptions of distance counseling and telemental health practice and training. *The Journal of Counselor Preparation and Supervision, 14*(3). https://digitalcommons.sacredheart.edu/jcps/vol14/iss3/3/

Salama, R. & Hinton, T. (2023). Online higher education: Current landscape and future trends. *Journal of Further and Higher Education, 47*(7), 913–924. https://doi.org/10.1080/0309877X.2023.2200136

Sampson, J. P., & Lenz, J. G. (2023). *Designing and implementing career interventions* (2nd ed.). National Career Development Association.

Sanford, N. (1967). *Where colleges fail: A study of the student as a person.* Jossey-Bass

Savickas, M. L., & Hartung, P. J. (2012). Career construction interview. http://www.vocopher.com/CSI/CCI.pdf

Schaffer, C. T., Nakrani, P., & Pirraglia, P. A. (2020). Telemental health care: A review of efficacy and interventions. *Telehealth and Medicine Today, 5*(4). https://doi.org/10.30953/tmt.v5.218

Shafer, S. P., & Clawson, T.W. (2007). The distance credentialed counselor. In J. F. Malone, R. M. Miller, & G. R. Walz, (Eds.). *Distance counseling: Expanding the counselor's reach and impact* (pp. 37–52). Counseling Outfitters.

Sheperis, D., & Sadeh-Sharvit, S. (2023). Using AI-supported supervision in a university telemental health training clinic. *Journal of Technology in Education and Supervision, 4,* Article 3. https://doi.org/10.61888/2692-4129.1093

Sherman, W. R., & Craig, A. B. (2018). *Understanding virtual reality: Interface, application, and design*. Elsevier Science.

Simms, D. C., Gibson, K., & O'Donnell, S. (2011). To use or not to use: Clinicians' perceptions of telemental health. *Canadian Psychology, 52*(1), 41–51. https://doi.org/10.1037/a0022275

Singh, A. A., Brandee, B., & Trepal, H. (2020). Using multicultural and social justice counseling competencies to decolonize counseling practice: The important roles of theory, power, and action. *Journal of Counseling & Development, 98,* 261–271. https://doi.org/10.1002/jcad.12321

Smith, T., Norton, A. M., & Marroquin, L. (2021). Virtual family play therapy: A clinician's guide to using directed family play therapy in telemental health. *Contemporary Family Therapy, 45*(1), 106–116. https://doi.org/10.1007/s10591-021-09612-7

Smith, R. L. (2015). *Treatment strategies for substance and process addictions.* American Counseling Association.

Soria, K. M., & Horgos, B. (2021). Factors associated with college students' mental health during the COVID-19 pandemic. *Journal of College Student Development, 62*(2), 236–242.

Sparks, K. (2021, March 21). *The Trevor Project launches new AI tool to support Crisis Counselor training.* https://www.thetrevorproject.org/blog/the-trevor-project-launches-new-ai-tool-to-support-crisis-counselor-training/

Stephan, S., Lever, N., Bernstein, L., Edwards, S., & Pruitt, D. (2016). Telemental health in schools. *Journal of Child and Adolescent Psychopharmacology, 26*(3), 266–272. https://doi.org/10.1089/cap.2015.0019

Stoller, E. (2019, March 28). Online education—the forgotten frontier in student affairs. *Inside Higher Ed.* https://www.insidehighered.com/blogs/student-affairs-and-technology/online-education-forgotten-frontier-student-affairs

Stretch, L.S., Nagel, D.M & Anthony, K (2013). Ethical framework for the use of technology in supervision. *Therapeutic Innovations in Light of Technology, 3*(2) 39–45. https://www.onlinetherapyinstitute.com/ethical-framework-technology-supervision/

Sue, D.W., Sue, D., Neville, H. A., & Smith, L. (2023). *Counseling the culturally diverse: Theory and practice* (9th ed.). Wiley.

Substance Abuse Mental Health Services Administration. (n.d.). https://www.samhsa.gov/

Sunderji, N., Crawford, A., & Jovanovic, M. (2014). Telepsychiatry in graduate medical education: A narrative review. *Academic Psychiatry, 39,* 55–62. https://doi.org/10.1007/s40596-014-0176-x

Tinto, V. (1987). *Leaving College.* University of Chicago Press.

Tozini, K., & Castiello-Gutiérrez, S. (2022). COVID-19 and international students: Examining perceptions of social support, financial well-being, psychological stress, and university response. *Journal of College Student Development, 63*(2), 134–150. https://doi.org/10.1353/csd.2022.0011

Trafton, A. (2018, December 13). Ingestible capsule can be controlled wirelessly. *MIT News.* https://news.mit.edu/2018/ingestible-pill-controlled-wirelessly-bluetooth-1213

Trepal, H., Haberstroh, S., Duffey, T., & Evans, M. (2007). Considerations and strategies for teaching online counseling skills: Establishing relationships in cyberspace. *Counselor Education & Supervision, 46*, 266–279. https://doi.org/10.1002/j.1556-6978.2007.tb00031.x

U. S. Bureau of Labor Statistics. (2019, April 17). *BLS history*. https://www.bls.gov/bls/history/timeline.htm

U.S. Department of Civil Rights. Americans with Disabilities Act. (2022, March 18). *Guidance on web accessibility and the ADA*. https://www.ada.gov/resources/web-guidance/

U.S. Department of Education. (2021). *Family Educational Rights and Privacy Act*. https://www2.ed.gov/policy/gen/guid/fpco/ferpa/index.html

U.S. Department of Education. (2023, May 16). *GEN-23-03: Requirements and responsibilities for third-party servicers and institutions*. https://fsapartners.ed.gov/knowledge-center/library/dear-colleague-letters/2023-02-15/requirements-and-responsibilities-third-party-servicers-and-institutions-updated-may-16-2023

U.S. Department of Health and Human Services. (n.d.). *Summary of the HIPAA privacy rule*. https://www.hhs.gov/hipaa/for-professionals/privacy/laws-regulations/index.html

U.S. Department of Health and Human Services. (2024). *Telehealth resources for providers*. https://telehealth.hhs.gov/providers

U.S. Department of Health and Human Services. (2020). *COVID-19 and HIPAA Bulletin: Limited waiver of HIPAA sanctions and penalties during nationwide national public health emergency*. https://www.hhs.gov/sites/default/files/hipaa-and-covid-19-limited-hipaa-waiver-bulletin-508.pdf

University of Maine. (n.d.). *Office of Research Compliance. Using social media for research purposes*. https://umaine.edu/research-compliance/human-subjects/social-media-guidance/

Viano, A. (2023, July 28). What is third-party risk, and what can higher education do about it? *Ed Tech: Focus on Higher Education*. https://edtechmagazine.com/higher/article/2023/07/what-third-party-risk-and-what-can-higher-education-do-about-it-perfcon

Villares, E., Starrett, A., & Limberg, D. (2022). Exploring school counseling during the first wave of COVID-19. *Journal of Counseling & Development, 100*(4), 386–398. https://doi.org/10.1002/jcad.12433

Wells, K. (2023, June 09). An eating disorder chatbot offered dieting advice, raising fears about AI in health. *National Public Radio*. https://www.npr.org/sections/health-shots/2023/06/08/1180838096/

an-eating-disorders-chatbot-offered-dieting-advice-raising-fears-about-ai-in-hea

Westra, K. (2018, October 28). Online student services: What, where, when, who, how, and most importantly why. *Educause Review.* https://er.educause.edu/articles/2018/10/online-student-services-what-where-who-when-how-and-most-importantly-why

Weintraub, E., Greenblatt, A. D., Chang, J., Himelhoch, S., & Welsh, C. (2018). Expanding access to Buprenorphine treatment in rural areas with use of telemedicine. *The American Journal of Addiction Studies, 27,* 612–617. https://doi.org/10.1111/ajad.12805

Weiss, B. J., Azevedo, K., Webb, K., Gimeno, J., & Cloitre, M. (2018). Telemental health delivery of Skills Training in Affective and Interpersonal Regulation (STAIR) for rural women veterans who have experienced military sexual trauma. *Journal of Traumatic Stress, 31,* 620–625. https://doi.org/10.1002/jts.22305

Whiston, S. C. (2017). *Principles and applications of assessment in counseling* (5th ed.). Cengage Learning.

Whittingham, M., & Martin, J. (2020, April). How to do group therapy using telehealth. American Psychological Association. https://www.apaservices.org/practice/legal/technology/group-therapy-telehealth-covid-19

World Health Organization. (2022). *Consolidated telemedicine implementation guide.* https://www.who.int/publications/i/item/9789240059184

World Health Organization and International Telecommunications Union. (2022). *WHO-ITU global standard for accessibility of telehealth services.* https://www.who.int/publications/i/item/9789240050464

Wright, A. J., Mihura, J. L., Pade, H., & McCord, D. M. (2020, May 1). *Guidance on psychological tele-assessment during the COVID-19 crisis.* American Psychological Association. https://www.apaservices.org/practice/reimbursement/health-codes/testing/tele-assessment-covid-19

Wu, Y., Fenfen, E., Wang, Y., Xu, M., Liu, S., Zhou, L., Song, G., Shang, X., Yang, C., Yang, K., & Li, X. (2023). Efficacy of internet-based cognitive behavioral therapy for depression in adolescents: A systematic review and meta-analysis. *Internet Interventions, 34,* Article 100673. https://doi.org/10.1016/j.invent.2023.100673

Zeligmari, M., Jones, J. L., Ataga, J., & McNiece, Z. P. (2022). Discrimination, social media use, and chronic stress in Black

Americans. *Journal of Mental Health Counseling, 44*(4), 327–342. https://doi.org/10.17744/mehc.44.4.04

Zimba, O., & Gasparyan, A. Y. (2021). Social media platforms: a primer for researchers. *Reumatologia, 59*(2), 68–72. https://doi.org/10.5114/reum.2021.102707

Glossary

AImorosexuality (also *IAmorosexuality*): The personal, emotional, or sexual attraction to artificial intelligence-generated content (Albalat Peraita, 2023).

Andragogy: "The art and science of helping adults learn," distinguishing it from *pedagogy*, which focuses on the teaching of children (Knowles, 1975).

Apps: see **Mobile apps**.

Assistive technology (AT): Products, equipment, and systems that enhance learning, working, and daily living for persons with disabilities.

Artificial intelligence (AI): The National Artificial Intelligence Act of 2020 (H.R. 6216) defines AI as "a machine-based system that can, for a given set of human-defined objectives, make predictions, recommendations, or decisions influencing real or virtual environments" (U.S. House of Representatives, 2020, Section 3, para. 3). AI can be utilized to generate content (written text, images, video), and mimic or predict human-like responses.

Asynchronous: Services (e.g., counseling, communication, instruction) are conducted in delayed time, with the parties (e.g., counselor, client, student, teacher) responding to messages at any point in time. More specifically, communication goes in one direction at a time, such as text messages, emails, photos, files, or videos created and sent to the recipient. The recipient may receive these messages immediately or retrieve them later (Myers & Turey, 2013).

Avatars (also *digital avatars*): A digital/virtual representation of a human being or fictional character that interacts with the technology user via speech, movement, or other life-like characteristics.

Blended platforms: Combines both synchronous and asynchronous services. Blended systems combine modalities such as chat, email, and video conferencing; may allow counselors to conduct TMH services while also including billing, appointment scheduling, and notes features.

Broadband (also *broadband internet, broadband speed*): Most easily defined as a high-speed internet connection that enables the rapid transfer of data and streaming content, such as live video conferencing.

Breakout rooms: A feature within most videoconferencing platforms, allowing the meeting organizer to assign smaller groups of attendees into virtual rooms and permitting small group meetings within a larger videoconference meeting.

Business associate: Business associates (also known as "third party vendors") consist of any outside party, program, and/or software used to conduct business beyond the client and counselor, agency, and/or organization. Business associates may include physical vendors (e.g., copy services, shipping services), yet in the case of telemental health, most often refer to digital support services, such as email or file store software systems, turnkey platforms, videoconferencing software, telephone service providers, or billing software or other products.

Business Associate Agreement (BAA): The BAA is a written agreement/statement between third-party vendors and the counselor/agency/organization detailing their data security and encryption practices, as well as HIPAA protections and the protection of PHI/e-PHI.

Chat (also *online chat*): Communication of short messages over the internet that typically occur within a specific software system (e.g., videoconferencing platform, gaming platform, mobile app, etc.). Like text messages (sent via mobile phone providers), chat messages are typically short and use truncated communication patterns. While chat messages are sent in "live" time, they can be read by the recipient at a later date/time.

Counseling Compact: An interstate compact in the U.S. allowing counselors licensed and residing in one state to apply for the privilege to practice in another state with minimal barriers and reduced costs. For more information, visit https://counselingcompact.org/.

Data mining: The National Institute of Standards and Technology (NIST), a division of the U.S. Department of Commerce, defines data mining as "an analytical process that attempts to find correlations or patterns in large data sets for the purpose of data or knowledge discovery" (U.S. Department of Commerce, NIST, 2020, p. 428).

Digisexuality: "People whose primary sexual identity comes through the use of technology" (McArthur & Twist, 2017, p. 334).

Digital divide: The National Digital Inclusion Alliance (NDIA) defines the digital divide as "the gap between those who have affordable access, skills, and support to engage online effectively and those who do not" (NDIA, n.d., para. 5).

Digital footprint: A trail of data that users create when posting online (Johnson, 2021).

Electronic medical records (EMR): Also known as *electronic health records*, an electronic record of a patient's medical history and treatment maintained over time. EMRs may be maintained through in-house programs or via third-party vendor software.

Electronic protected health information (ePHI): Creating, maintaining, or receiving protected health information (see **PHI**) in electronic form (U.S. Department of Health and Human Services, n.d.).

Emojis/emoticons: Symbols or images within certain software programs that allow users to portray emotion or other words via pictures; emoticons, the precursor to emojis, were typically composed of common keyboard characters (e.g., punctuation marks, letters, numbers) arranged to form images. Both are regularly utilized in text and chat communication.

Encryption: The process of changing plain digital text to cipher text to prevent anyone but the intended party from receiving or interpreting digital information.

Face-to-face (also *F2F* or *f2f*): Counseling service performed in a live, in-person setting. Note that online synchronous services are typically considered TMH services, not F2F services.

Family Educational Rights and Privacy Act (FERPA): Federal law protecting students' educational records (U.S. Department of Education, 2021)

Health Insurance Portability and Accountability Act (HIPAA): A "set of national standards for the protection of certain health information" (U.S. Department of Health and Human Services, n.d., para. 1).

Health Professional Shortage Areas (HPSA): The Health Resources and Services Administration (HRSA), a division of the U.S. Department of Health and Human Services, maintains a data warehouse and dashboard of HPSAs in health care, dental care, and mental health care. As of January 2023, 158 million people live in mental health care provider shortage areas (HRSA, 2023).

iCBT (also known as "internet-based CBT"): Uses a digital platform to deliver cognitive behavioral therapy (CBT) in different formats, including blended, guided, and unguided delivery; may include interactive components such as games, videos, and assignments (Wu et al., 2023).

Internet Protocol (IP) Address: An individual identifier for each computer/device that transmits information over a computer network, which supports user identification and location.

Learning Management System (LMS): A software system that allows educational institutions and organizations to manage educational, training, and learning environments (e.g., Canvas, Blackboard). An LMS is used to organize instruction, make learning more engaging, and serve as a repository for information (e.g., student/instructor files, assignments, links to external platforms, videos).

Lurkers: People who linger or remain ("lurk") in online groups or discussions without participating; lurkers may be seen as observers but may also disrupt group member trust and cohesion.

Mobile apps: "Mobile apps (mobile applications; apps): software designed for use on small, wireless devices such as smartphones or tablets, rather than desktop or laptop computers. Apps may be affiliated with a corresponding website or may be a standalone app without a computer based counterpart." (SAP, n.d., para. 1).

Modality: The medium through which counselors deliver counseling. Prevalent counseling modalities include telephone, email, text, chat, and videoconferencing, or F2F. It is expected that variations of these modalities, if not entirely new modalities, will emerge in the future.

Multifactor Authentication (or Two-Factor Authentication, 2FA): A technological security measure requiring the user to enter at least two points of data/evidence/authentication to access the system, as opposed to a single sign-on (e.g., password) to access the technology.

Poster: Someone who posts regularly on online mediums, such as chats, discussion boards, or other forums. Posters may be active, healthy participants or dominate discussions in a way that disregards other members.

Platforms: The context in which TMH services occur, including primarily **synchronous**, **asynchronous**, **blended**, and **turnkey** services. It is expected that variations of these platforms, if not entirely new types, will emerge in the future.

Privacy settings: Settings on software systems, internet browsers, and mobile apps allow users to control the amount of data visible to the public or within identified networks.

Protected Health Information (PHI): Individually identified health information, including demographic data, relating to past, present, or future physical or mental health conditions, provision of health care, or past/present/future payment for provision of health care) (U.S. Department of Health and Human Services, n.d., para. 13-14).

Screen sharing: A feature within most videoconferencing platforms that allows a user to share their computer or device screen with other members of the videoconference meeting, allowing the user to share documents, videos, or other on-screen images with all parties.

Smartphones: Smartphones are communication devices containing an operating system that provides many of the same features as a computer, including internet access, mobile apps, and video streaming, as opposed to traditional mobile or cell phones that provide basic phone and text services only.

Social media: Internet websites and mobile apps that allow individuals to post content and participate in social networking

Synchronous: Synchronous services, such as telephone conversations or video-conferencing sessions, that occur in real-time. More specifically, synchronous services allow communication to go in both directions during the exchange or multiple directions in the case of group counseling or classroom instruction simultaneously (Myers & Turvey, 2013).

Teledildonics: The use of internet technology to control or operate the use of sex toys between two users (Knowles, 2017). Other terms include "dildonics," "cyber-dildonics," and "smart sex toys."

Texting, text messaging (text-talk): The sending of short messages consisting of alpha and numeric characters, traditionally via mobile phones or smartphones; text communication patterns (e.g., text-talk) include short messages, abbreviations or acronyms, and emojis/emoticons.

Turnkey platforms. Platforms that provide a blended platform, network of providers, and pool of potential clients.

Two-Factor Authentication: see **Multifactor authentication.**

Videoconferencing: Meetings that occur via platforms that enable audio and video to be shared in real-time (synchronous). The number of people participating in videoconference meetings may be limited by the software or meeting settings. Other terms include "video meetings" or "video sessions."

Wearable technology: Includes any device that monitors physical functioning and records the data, storing it in a remote location (e.g., cloud storage). Examples include smart watches, which monitor sleep, exercise, and breathing, as well as alcohol-use ankle monitors.

Zoom bombers: People who join online meetings or groups (including phone, video, or chat/discussion board) with the purpose of disrupting the meeting; examples include people who use disparaging, discriminatory, or disturbing language, images, or videos to disrupt the group.

Index

A

Academic journals, 8, 137
Journal of Technology in Counseling Education and Supervision (JTCES), 8
The Journal of Telemedicine (TJT), 8
Telehealth and Medicine Today (THMT), 8
Addictions counseling, 16, 71, 89, 113, 124, 145-159, 189. See also Substance use disorder
abstinence and harm reduction, 147, 149, 151
clients under the influence, 150
ethical and legal concerns, 148–149, 152, 157
online assessment, 152–155
process addictions, 145, 151–152
sample lessons, 152–159
TMH benefits and challenges, 149–150
teaching techniques, 150–152
Addiction Severity Index (ASI), 124–125
Adolescents. See Children and adolescents
Adult education. See Andragogy
Affinity groups, 43, 57, 210
Alcoholics Anonymous (AA). See Self-help groups
Alcohol Use Disorders Identification Test (AUDIT), 113, 153. See also Substance use disorders
American Academy of Pediatrics (AAP), 55, 58
American Association for Marriage and Family Therapy (AAMFT), 221–222. See also Family counseling. See also Marriage counseling
American Association of Sexuality Educators, Counselors and Therapists (AASECT), 55. See also Sexuality and technology
American Counseling Association (ACA), 7, 24
ACA Code of Ethics, 7, 24–28, 30–32, 34, 58, 74, 88, 99, 105–108, 117–118, 124, 133, 136–137, 139, 141, 149–150, 157, 165, 180, 196, 221–222, 279–283
Governing Council, 41
American Educational Research Association (AERA), 118–119. See also Research
The Standards for Educational and Psychological Testing, 118
American Mental Health Counselors Association (AMHCA), 4–7, 100, 118, 133, 176, 180, 264. See also Clinical mental health counseling
Standards of Practice for Clinical Mental Health Counseling, 4
Technology Supported Counseling and Communications (TSCC), 4–6, 176, 180

American Psychiatric Association (APA), 3, 180–181
APA App Evaluation Model (App Advisor), 181, 273
American School Counselor Association (ASCA), 4, 7, 100, 118, 133, 229–230, 233, 235–236, 240, 264. See also School counseling
ASCA Ethical Standards, 237, 240–241
American Society of Addiction Medicine (ASAM), 113. See also Addictions counseling
ASAM Criteria Assessment Interview, 113
Americans with Disabilities Act (ADA), 192, 194–196, 211, 261. See also Disabilities
American Telemedicine Association (ATA), 7
Andragogy, 17–18, 28, 43, 57, 73, 90, 103, 118, 130, 133, 150, 164, 179, 196, 210, 221, 235, 266, 309
Antisocial personality disorder (APD), 185–187
Artificial intelligence (AI), 89, 105–106, 132, 164, 257, 271–273
AImorosexuality, 59, 191, 309. See also Sexuality and technology
avatars, 272, 275, 309
Freed.AI, 271
generative pretrained transformer (GPT), 271
ChatGPT, 105–107, 135–138, 164, 166, 271
OpenAI, 271
Assessment and diagnostic processes, 113–118, 175, 180–183
ethical codes, 118
online assessments, 116–118
interpreting results, 118–119
proctored administration, 117–120
psychometric properties, 119–122
test environment, 117–118
sample lessons, 120–126
teaching techniques, 118–120
Assistive technology. See Disabilities
Assistive Technology Industry Association (ATIA), 196
Association for Addiction Professionals. See NAADAC
Association for Assessment and Research in Counseling (AARC), 122. See also Assessment and diagnostic processes. See also Research
AARC Assessment Database, 122
Association for Specialists in Group Work (ASGW), 99, 101. See also Group work
Guiding Principles for Group Work, 99, 105–107
Ten Tips for the Facilitation of Virtual Groups, 101
Asynchronous services. See Platforms

B

Ball Tran, Kami, 226–228
Bandwidth, 44, 89. See also Broadband
Ben-Porath, Yossef S., 117, 119
Bethea, James, 60–62, 167–168
Blumer, Markie L., 290
Books. See also Suggested reading
Dictionary of Occupational Titles, 73
Distance Counseling: Expanding the Counselor's Reach and Impact, 7
Mental Measurements Yearbook (MMY), 121
Tests in Print, 121
Occupational Outlook Handbook, 73, 163
Borenstein, Lynn, 221

Brain development, 59
Breadwinner's Institute, 69
Broadband, 42–44, 309. See also Bandwidth
Brott, Pamelia, 75–79
Brown, Duane, 69, 167
Brown-Smythe, Claudette, 79–83, 236–241
Business Associate Agreement (BAA), 25, 28, 88, 131, 210, 310

C

CACREP Standards, 8, 12–13, 53, 145, 175–176, 190, 205, 235, 248–251, 255–256. See also Council for Accreditation of Counseling and Related Educational Programs
  Addictions Counseling, 146–148
  Assessment and Diagnostic Processes, 114–116
  Career Counseling, 161–163
  Career Development, 70–71
  Clinical Mental Health Counseling, 176–178, 230–233
  Clinical Rehabilitation Counseling, 190–192
  College Counseling and Student Affairs, 206–208
  Counseling Practice and Relationships, 85–88
  Doctoral Counseling, 256–257
  Doctoral Leadership and Advocacy, 264–266
  Doctoral Research and Scholarship, 261–264
  Doctoral Supervision, 257–259
  Doctoral Teaching, 259–261
  Group Counseling and Group Work, 100–101
  Lifespan Development, 54–55
  Marriage, Couple, and Family Counseling, 218–220
  Professional Counseling Orientation and Ethical Practice, 22–23
  Rehabilitation Counseling, 192–194
  Research and Program Evaluation, 130–131
  Social and Cultural Identities and Experiences, 39–41
Career Construction Interview (CCI), 165
Career counseling, 4, 71–73, 75, 161–164. See also Career development
  artificial intelligence (AI), 164
  asynchronous, 171–174. See also Platforms
  decision-making, 79–83, 167
  sample lessons, 79–83, 167–174
  teaching techniques, 164–166
Career development, 13, 69–73, 161, 164. See also Career counseling
  artificial intelligence (AI), 164
  college information, 79
  decision-making, 79–83
  online career information, 13, 73–75, 79–82
  sample lessons, 75–83
  teaching techniques, 73–75
  transformational learning, 75–79
Career planning services. See Career development
Case studies, 28, 58, 74, 140, 222
Center for Connected Health Policy (CCHP), 6
Center for Credentialing and Education (CCE), 7, 13, 172. See also Credentialing
Centers for Disease Control and Prevention (CDC), 5
Certified rehabilitations counselors (CRCs), 189, 199. See also Clinical rehabilitation counseling
ChatGPT. See Artificial intelligence

Children and adolescents, 17, 26–27, 31, 56–58, 61, 180–181, 239, 253. See also Family counseling
play therapy, 221
screen time, 58
Cicco, Gina, 139–141, 241–244
Client confidentiality. See Confidentiality
Clinical mental health counseling (CMHC), 175–179, 189, 230
advocacy, 178, 264
co-occurring disorders, 180
diagnostic criteria, 180–183
safety planning, 179–181
sample lessons, 181–187
teaching techniques, 179–181
treatment planning, 181–184, 187
Clinical rehabilitation counseling, 145, 189–196
accessibility, 194–197
sample lessons, 198–203
teaching techniques, 196–197
technology compliance, 195–196, 211
Cognitive behavioral therapy (CBT), 87, 97, 183, 311
Collaborative care, 181, 197, 202–203
College and student affairs counseling, 4, 161, 205–208
delivery services, 211–213
distance services, 206–212, 215–216
online policies, 210–211, 214
sample lessons, 211–216
student engagement, 209, 211
teaching techniques, 209–211
Commission on Rehabilitation Counselor Certification (CRCC), 100, 189. See also Clinical rehabilitation counseling
Commission on Rehabilitation Education (CORE), 189. See also Clinical rehabilitation counseling
Community Technical Assistance Center of New York (CTACNY), 101
Confidentiality, 16, 25, 32, 46–47, 85, 97–98, 102–104, 118, 125, 150, 152, 221, 238, 241, 253, 257, 272–273. See also Data safety and security. See also Health Insurance Portability and Accountability Act
Conners Rating Scale, 113. See also Assessment and diagnostic processes
Corey, David M., 117, 119
Council for Accreditation of Counseling and Related Educational Programs (CACREP), 8–9, 12–13, 17, 21, 30–31, 53, 76, 103, 145, 156, 161, 176, 189, 218, 247, 275
Foundational Counseling Curriculum, 19–141, 145, 161, 175–176. See also CACREP Standards
Council for the Advancement of Standards in Higher Education (CAS), 210, 215–216
Counseling Compact, 23, 29, 41, 44, 50, 177–178, 268
Counseling Outfitters, 7
Counseling practice. See Counseling relationships. See Professional practice
Counseling relationships, 27, 29–31, 42, 57, 85–90, 102, 221. See also Ethical practice
online communication, 89–90
sample lessons, 92–98
teaching techniques, 90–91
virtual relationships, 24, 74
Counselor Activity Self Efficacy Scales (CASES), 252
Counselor education and supervision (CES), 8, 13–14, 247–252, 255–266
CACREP curriculum standards, 255–256

doctoral counseling, 256–257
doctoral leadership and advocacy, 264–266
doctoral research and scholarship, 261–264
doctoral supervision, 257–259
doctoral teaching, 259–261
teaching techniques, 266–268
Counselors-in-training (CITs), 9, 13–14, 16–18, 22, 24, 27, 31, 39, 41–42, 53–54, 57, 69, 73, 85, 99–103, 113–114, 117–118, 129, 146, 163–164, 176, 178–179, 190, 195, 205, 217, 229, 234, 247–253, 255–257, 259, 262, 264, 274, 275–276
Couple counseling. See Marriage counseling
COVID-19 pandemic, 3–4, 8, 11–13, 17, 24, 56, 69, 148–149, 199, 202, 208, 220–221, 229, 234, 247, 266, 269–270, 272
Craig, Alan B., 270
Credentialing, 7, 28, 33–37, 72, 165–166
Board Certified TeleMental Health Provider (BC-TMH), 7–8, 23
Distance Certified Counselor (DCC), 8, 13
Distance Counselor Certification (DCC), 13
Distance Counseling Credential (DCC), 7

D

Data mining, 274–276
Data safety and security, 28, 31, 73, 85, 89, 97–98, 117–118, 124, 132–134, 148, 157, 179–181, 197, 203, 209–210, 214, 221, 223, 236–238, 240, 249, 252–253, 272–273, 274, 277, 280–283. See also Confidentiality
automated services, 209–210
encryption, 15, 25, 28, 31, 36, 44, 86, 88, 116, 124, 133, 148, 157, 177, 179. 214, 220–221, 236, 238, 252, 311
multifactor authentication, 14, 312
privacy settings, 25–27, 117–118, 199, 237–238, 240, 249, 312
third-party software, 28, 132, 134, 195, 209–210, 214, 236, 272, 274
Diagnostic processes. See Assessment and diagnostic processes
Digital divide, 42–43, 178, 310
Digital footprint, 16, 56, 310
Disabilities, 26, 43, 49–50, 56, 76, 113, 189, 195, 200, 202–203, 209–210, 282. See also Americans with Disabilities Act
assistive technology (AT), 195–196, 309
people with disabilities (PWD), 41, 55–56, 189–196
web accessibility, 195–196
Diversity. See Social and cultural diversity
Doctoral research. See Research

E

Electromyography (EMG), 184
Electronic medical records (EMR), 87–88, 178, 192, 271–272, 310–311
Email counseling. See Platforms
Emergency situations, 88–89, 101, 148, 176, 179, 238
duty to warn, 29
emergency contacts, 29, 31, 90–91, 107, 176, 179
procedures in fieldwork, 252–253
Erford, Bradley T., 139, 141
Erikson, Erik, 58

Eschenauer, Robert, 181–184
Ethical practice, 7, 12, 15, 18, 21–27, 72, 76, 99–100, 102, 129, 149, 179, 206, 209, 251, 275
  informed consent, 27–31
  sample lessons, 29–37
  teaching techniques, 28–29

F

Face-to-face (F2F) counseling, 11, 13–14, 21, 27, 76, 85, 88, 102–103, 145, 148, 165, 179, 186, 189, 218, 260, 273, 311
Family counseling, 217–221. See also Marriage counseling
  challenges, 221, 227
  genogram tools, 220, 223
  impact of technology, 222
  mock family sessions, 222
  sample lessons, 223–228
  teaching techniques, 221–223
  TMH guidelines, 220–222, 227
  translating theories, 223
Family Educational Rights and Privacy Act (FERPA), 236–238, 240, 311
Federal laws. See Licensing and laws
Fieldwork, 11, 18, 247–253. See also Professional practice
  CACREP curricular standards, 248–251
    communication with supervisors, 250–251
    program administration, 248–249
    seminar instruction, 249–250
  recordings, 249, 252
  techniques, 251–253
  vlogging, 252
Foundational Counseling Curriculum. See Council for Accreditation of Counseling and Related Educational Programs

G

Gamblers Anonymous (GA). See Self-help groups
Gasparyan, Armen Yuri, 133
Global Career Development Facilitator (GCDF), 172. See also Career development
Gonzalez, Leo, 152–155
Goss, Stephen, 252
Group counseling, 15, 99–103, 149, 249
  engaging group members, 102–103, 105
  facilitating online groups, 101–104, 107–111
  online attacks, 108–111
  sample lessons, 105–111
  teaching techniques, 103–105
Group work, 99–100. See also Group counseling. See also Self-help groups

H

Harrichand, John J. S., 29–32
Hazel, Cameka, 79–83, 236–241
Health and Human Services. See U.S. Department of Health and Human Services
Health Insurance Portability and Accountability Act (HIPAA), 11, 28, 148, 221, 236–238, 240, 273, 311. See also Confidentiality. See also Data safety and security
  electronic protected health information (ePHI), 148, 310–311
  protected health information (PHI), 310, 312
Health professional shortage areas (HPSA), 23, 40, 43–44, 178
Health Resources and Services Administration (HRSA), 6, 43
Hertlein, Katherine M., 220, 222
Hunter, Daniel, 102

I

Informed consent, 27–28, 31, 132, 179, 221, 253, 280, 283, 285
sample lesson, 105–106
Institutional Review Boards (IRBs), 133, 263
Intake. See Screening and intake
International Association of Addictions and Offender Counselors (IAAOC), 149. See also Addictions counseling
International Association of Marriage and Family Counselors (IAMFC), 221–222. See also Family counseling. See also Marriage counseling
International Telecommunication Union (ITU), 5
Internet protocol (IP) addresses, 132, 311

J

Jalilzadeh, Nouna, 105–108, 135–139
Jones, Michael, 48–51
Journals. See Academic journals

K

Knowle, Malcolm, 17–18, 130
Krach, S. Kathleen, 116, 122

L

Learning management systems (LMS), 14, 16, 48, 92, 94, 106, 136, 139, 140, 242, 311. See also Videoconferencing
LGBTQ+ community, 31–32, 43, 49, 208, 210, 276
The Trevor Project, 276
Licensing and laws, 17, 50, 148, 163, 165, 205, 229, 249, 274
federal, 148, 150, 196, 249
sample lesson, 33–37
state, 4, 28, 31–32, 34, 44, 71–72, 99, 124, 148, 157, 164, 166, 249
multistate licensure, 29, 164
Li, Ming-hui, 45–47, 96–98
Lifespan development, 53–57
digital detox, 63–66
generational differences, 56ß
impact of technology, 53–55, 57–63, 65
sample lessons, 60–67
social-emotional wellness, 56–57
social media, 56–59, 67
teaching techniques, 57–59
Logistics, 90

M

Marriage counseling, 217–221, 275. See also Family counseling
challenges, 221
impact of technology, 222–223
mock couple sessions, 222
sample lessons, 223–228
TMH guidelines, 220–221
teaching techniques, 221–223
Medicaid, 6, 148, 178, 192, 220
Medicare, 41, 148, 178, 192, 220
Medication-assisted treatment (MAT), 147, 149, 151, 157–158, 202–203. See also Addictions counseling
Mental health counseling. See Clinical mental health counseling
Mental status exam (MSE), 89, 149, 180. See also Assessment and diagnostic processes
Minnesota Multiphasic Personality Inventory (MMPI), 121. See also Assessment and diagnostic processes
Minors. See Children and adolescents

Mobile apps, 179–181, 273–275. See also Smartphones
APA App Evaluation Model (App Advisor), 181, 273
sample lesson, 96–98
Modalities, 13–16, 18, 21, 29, 33, 46, 85, 90–95, 100, 104, 114, 117, 150–151, 180–181, 196–197, 218, 222, 225, 252, 259, 312. See also Platforms
apps. See Mobile apps
chat, 15, 62, 85, 90–93, 102, 104, 109–110, 168, 252
email, 16, 90–91, 168, 172–173
emojis/emoticons, 87, 90, 102, 311
text, 87–90, 131, 149, 179, 195–196, 252, 276
video, 5, 14–15, 42, 48, 56, 77, 89–95, 104, 140, 148, 157, 164, 179, 249, 252. See also Videoconferencing
Multicultural and Social Justice Counseling Competencies (MSJCC), 41–42. See also Multiculturalism
Multiculturalism, 26, 35, 39, 41, 43, 45–47, 49, 75, 82, 282. See also Social and cultural diversity

N

NAADAC, the Association for Addiction Professionals, 100, 118, 133, 148–150, 157, 264. See also Addictions counseling
Nadrich, Tyce, 92–95
Narcotics Anonymous (NA). See Self-help groups
NASPA, Student Affairs Administrators in Higher Education, 205. See also College and student affairs counseling
National Association of Student Personnel Administrators. See NASPA
National Board for Certified Counselors (NBCC), 4–5, 12–13
NBCC Code of Ethics, 26–28, 30–32, 58, 88, 279, 283–286
Standards for the Ethical Practice of WebCounseling (1997), 13
National Career Development Association (NCDA), 4, 7, 72, 74, 121, 100, 163, 165. See also Career development
A Comprehensive Guide to Career Assessment, 121
National Certification Commission for Addiction Professionals (NCC AP), 149. See also Addictions counseling
National Eating Disorders Association (NEDA), 272
National Employment Counseling Association (NECA), 74, 165. See also Career counseling. See also Career Development
National Institute of Mental Health (NIMH), 5. See also Clinical mental health counseling
National Public Radio (NPR), 272

O

O'Hagan, Joni, 211–213
On-campus classroom instruction, 14
Overeaters Anonymous (OA). See Self-help groups

P

Parsons, Frank, 69
Paulino, Rosa Aleida, 208–209
Perepiczka, Michelle, 223–228
PESI (continuing education), 7, 12
Pew Research Center, 42, 132
Phillips, Melissa Lee, 132–133
Piaget, Jean, 58

PICCA Model, 242–243. See also School counseling
Platforms, 12, 14, 34, 36, 48, 56–57, 82, 89, 195, 208, 238, 274, 312. See also Learning Management Systems. See also Modalities. See also Social media
asynchronous services, 14, 77, 90, 102, 168, 221, 225, 312
asynchronous career counseling, 171–174
online asynchronous classroom instruction, 14–15, 48–50, 93, 106, 121–122, 124, 126, 136, 153, 156, 158–159, 171–174, 187, 198, 200, 202–203, 212, 216, 275
email counseling, 14, 16, 89, 149, 168
blended platforms, 309, 312
internet-based cognitive behavioral therapy (iCBT), 87, 311
synchronous services, 14, 34, 77–78, 102, 221, 225, 312
breakout rooms, 15, 62, 141, 153, 212, 216, 243–244, 310
online synchronous classroom instruction, 14–15, 30, 45, 48–49, 62, 64, 93, 96, 105–106, 109, 121–122, 124, 126, 136, 140, 153, 156, 158, 167–168, 173, 186, 198, 200, 202–203, 212, 216, 242, 267, 275
turnkey platforms, 14, 28, 88, 312–313
Pogoda, Terri K., 195
Posttraumatic stress disorder (PTSD), 178, 270
Prioleau, Brittany L., 63–66
Priya, Lakshmi G. G., 270
Professional counseling. See Career counseling
Professional ethics. See Ethical practice
Professional orientation, 21–23, 250
Professional practice, 8–9, 90, 247–253. See also Fieldwork
CACREP curricular standards, 248–251
communication with supervisors, 250–251
program administration, 248–249
seminar instruction, 249–250
fieldwork techniques, 251–253
Program evaluation, 129–133, 261. See also Research
sample lessons, 135–138
teaching techniques, 133–135
Public Health Institute (PHI), 6

R

Raja, M., 270
Ready Minds, 7, 13
Rehabilitation counseling. See Clinical rehabilitation counseling
Rehabilitation Engineering and Assistive Technology Society of North America (RESNA), 196. See also Clinical rehabilitation counseling
Relationships. See Counseling relationships
Research, 129–133, 256. See also Program evaluation
AI integration, 132, 135–139. See also Artificial intelligence
databases, 132, 134–136
doctoral research, 261–264, 267
online research tools, 132–135
open forums, 132–133
quantitative and qualitative, 130, 134–135, 139–141
sample lessons, 135–141

survey tools, 132–135
teaching techniques, 133–135
transcription services, 130, 135, 272
Rewa, Jeanne, 102
Robertson, Heather C., 90, 120–126, 156–159, 171–174, 198–203, 215–216

S

Sadeh-Sharvit, Shiri, 257
School counseling, 4, 71, 161, 229–234. See also College and student affairs counseling
academics, 229, 235
classroom guidance, 236, 241–243
college and career goals, 229, 236, 239
counselor wellness, 234. See also Self-care plan
decision-making, 236–241
parental consultations, 233, 235–236
sample lessons, 236–244
school policy, 233–234
teaching techniques, 234–236
tech awareness, 236–241
Screening and intake, 26, 31, 88, 90, 149, 153–154, 187, 229, 271–272. See also Assessment and diagnostic processes
career counseling intake, 165
Screen sharing. See Videoconferencing
Sears, Susan, 69
Self-care plan, 29, 268
Self-help groups, 103, 148–149, 151
Severe mental illness (SMI), 178
Sexuality and technology, 59
AImorosexuality, 59, 191, 309
digisexuality, 59, 191, 272, 310
teledildonics, 59, 191, 313
Sheperis, Donna, 257
Sherman, William R., 270
Shupp, Matthew R., 33–37
Smartphones, 42, 96–97, 273, 312. See also Mobile apps
Smith, Tiffany, 221
Sniatecki, Jessica L., 185–187
SOAP (subjective, objective, assessment, plan) format, 271
Social and cultural diversity, 35, 39–43, 49, 210. See also Affinity groups. See also Multiculturalism
directories and services, 48–51
sample lessons, 45–51
social justice, 35, 39, 41–42, 49
teaching techniques, 43–44
Social media, 4, 7, 24, 26, 28, 30–31, 74, 149–150, 221, 241, 279–281, 283, 285–286
open forums in online research, 132–134
social-emotional wellness, 56–59
Spellman, Qiana, 108–111
State laws. See Licensing and laws
Stretch, Loriann S., 252
Strong Interest Inventory (STRONG), 121. See also Assessment and diagnostic processes
Student affairs. See College and student affairs counseling
Student Affairs Administrators in Higher Education. See NASPA
Substance Abuse and Mental Health Services Administration (SAMHSA), 3, 5, 63, 150, 153. See also Addictions counseling. See also Substance use disorder
Substance Use Confidentiality Regulations, 150
Substance use disorder (SUD), 3, 63, 65, 124, 145, 148–149, 152, 154–155, 157, 180, 202–203. See also Addictions counseling
Suggested reading, 8–9, 185. See also Books

Supervision. See Counselor education and supervision
Survey tools. See Research
Synchronous services. See Platforms

T

Training, 7
Transcription services. See Research
Twelve-step groups. See Self-help groups
Twist, Markie L. C., 222

U

University of Rhode Island Change Assessment (URICA), 124, 157–158. See also Assessment and diagnostic processes
U.S. Bureau of Labor Statistics (BLS), 73–74, 132
U.S. Census Bureau, 44, 74
U.S. Department of Civil Rights, 195–196
U.S Department of Education, 209, 260
U.S. Department of Health and Human Services (HHS), 7, 11
U.S. Department of Veterans Affairs (VA), 195

V

Viano, Andy, 209
Videoconferencing, 12, 14–15, 28, 46, 56, 80, 89, 92, 139, 236, 274, 313
  screen sharing, 56, 74, 87, 109–110, 164, 179, 199, 312
Virtual reality (VR), 270–271, 273, 275–276
Virtual relationships. See Counseling relationships

W

Wearable technology, 87, 146, 148, 273, 313
Western Association for Counselor Education and Supervision (WACES), 8. See also Counselor education and supervision
Westra, Kayla, 208
World Health Organization (WHO), 5
Wright, A. Jordan, 118

Z

Zimba, Olena, 133
Zur Institute, 7

About the Author

Dr. Heather C. Robertson (she/her) is a Professor and the Chair of Counselor Education at St. John's University. She is a Licensed Professional Counselor (LPC, CT), Licensed Mental Health Counselor (LMHC, NY), Nationally Certified Counselor (NCC), Certified Rehabilitation Counselor (CRC), Credentialed Alcoholism and Substance Abuse Counselor (CASAC, NY), Approved Clinical Supervisor (ACS), Global Career Development Facilitator (GCDF), and Board Certified Telemental Health Provider (BC-TMH). She earned a PhD in Counselor Education & Supervision from Virginia Tech, and an MS in Counseling & Guidance from Texas A & M University at Corpus Christi. Research and advocacy efforts include College and Career Transition, Substance Abuse, Military and Veterans, Telemental Health, and reducing the stigma of Mental Illness and Addiction. She has been researching, publishing, and practicing in telemental health since 2016, having received national, regional, and local grants in her research. She is the author of *Telemental Health and Distance Counseling: A Counselor's Guide to Decisions, Resources, and Practice* (2021).